Vitamin K
and the Newborn

Dr Sara Wickham

Vitamin K and the Newborn
Second edition published 2017 by Birthmoon Creations
© 2017 Sara Wickham
www.sarawickham.com

Sara Wickham has asserted her moral right to be named as the author of this work in accordance with the Copyright, Designs and Patents Act of 1988.

ISBN-10: 1999806409
ISBN-13: 978-1-9998064-0-8
Also available as an e-book

Cover design by Sanyukta Stargazer
www.sanyuktastargazer.com

This book offers general information for interest only and does not constitute or replace individualised professional midwifery or medical care and advice. Whilst every effort has been made to ensure the accuracy and currency of the information herein, the author accepts no liability or responsibility for any loss or damage caused, or thought to be caused, by making decisions based upon the information in this book and recommends that you use it in conjunction with other trusted sources of information.

ABOUT THE AUTHOR

Dr Sara Wickham PhD, RM, MA, PGCert, BA(Hons) is a multi-passionate midwife, educator, writer and researcher who works independently, dividing her working time between speaking, writing, teaching online courses and live workshops, consulting and creating resources for midwives and birth workers.

Sara's career has been varied; she has lived and worked in the UK, the USA and New Zealand, edited three professional journals and lectured in more than twenty-five countries.

You can find Sara online at www.sarawickham.com, where she writes a twice weekly blog and a free monthly newsletter. Some of her work is also shared at www.facebook.com/saramidwife and @DrSaraWickham

Also by Sara Wickham

Anti-D in Midwifery: panacea or paradox?
Appraising Research into Childbirth
Birthing Your Placenta (with Nadine Edwards)
Group B Strep Explained
Inducing Labour: making informed decisions
Midwifery Best Practice (volumes 1-5)
Sacred Cycles: the spiral of women's wellbeing
101 Tips for planning, writing and surviving your dissertation

Acknowledgements

Most of the books that I have written owe their existence to women and families who asked me questions that I couldn't answer. I want to begin by thanking all of you, whether your questions are in the past, present or future. Your desire to seek out what is best for yourselves and your baby and your challenges to what are sometimes contradictory and illogical statements are responsible for important shifts in thinking in medical and maternity care. Special thanks to those who have shared their own stories in this book.

Books do take a village to raise, and I have been supported in bringing this one to reality by a fabulous team of midwives, birth activists, childbirth educators, doctors and friends. In particular, I want to thank Beverley Beech, Gill Boden, Julie Bullard, Jude Davis, Nadine Edwards, Julie Frohlich, Ina May Gaskin, Chris Hackforth, Jessie Johnson-Cash and Sally Marchant, who all helped it become better through their reading, comments, suggestions and advice.

During the writing process, I invited questions for the FAQ section via my website, www.sarawickham.com, and we received an unprecedented number of replies – thank you all. I have tried to answer all your questions, and I hope you will forgive me for amalgamating a few.

Perhaps most importantly, I'd like to thank the late Dr Edmund Hey, whose comments, work and willingness to dialogue helped to build an important bridge between those who approach this topic from different perspectives.

Contents

Introduction

I learned early on in my midwifery education that vitamin K was a vital, lifesaving substance. I was taught that it should be given to all newborn babies within a couple of hours of their birth, ideally by injection. It could also be given by mouth but the injection was considered to be better, because the drug would remain in the baby's system for longer and would be released slowly over time. I learned to explain to parents that vitamin K was necessary to prevent their baby from bleeding. The suggestion that their baby could bleed without vitamin K is enough to scare anyone into agreeing to its administration, but we were taught to explain other things too. So I learned to tell parents that all babies are born without the vitamin K that they need, which is why we administer it in the birthing room. Like all student midwives, I learned all of these 'facts' and I practised giving vitamin K injections safely and proficiently before documenting its administration in the medical notes.

And then I met Laura.

Laura (who, like all the parents that I'll refer to in this book, has been given a pseudonym to ensure confidentiality) was pregnant with her third baby. Her first two children had had vitamin K, as was considered normal, routine, usual practice, but she had always wondered why vitamin K was deemed necessary for all babies. Why, she asked, after millennia of human evolution, are all babies born without a vital substance?

Laura's questions were good ones, but at the time I didn't have good answers to them. Not for the last time in my midwifery career, questions posed by women and their families inspired trips to the library and made me question the things that I had been taught to believe and say. Laura's curiosity and research inspired my own; consequently my understanding and practice changed dramatically.

Over time I came to understand that, while vitamin K *is* a vital, life-saving substance, the story and the issues are more complex. As with any drug or intervention, vitamin K has potential downsides as well as benefits. As I met more families who questioned why they should let us inject a substance into their newly born baby, I found myself spending a good bit of time explaining the issues to parents and helping them work out which decision was the right one for them and their baby.

Having these long conversations has been easier for me than for many midwives because I have tended to work in settings where I can spend more time with people than some of my colleagues can. Some women don't even get to have a midwife or another trusted woman-centred person whom they can talk with about such issues and decisions, and that's one of the main reasons that this book came into being. If you are a parent, I am hoping that it will help you to better understand the evidence and the issues and be able to make the decision that is right for you and your baby. If you are a caregiver, I'm hoping it will help you better understand the debates and the evidence so that you can answer the questions that you might be asked.

The first edition of this book (Wickham 2003), published many years ago by the Association for Improvements in the Maternity Services (AIMS), was a slim booklet that just discussed the key elements of the decision. But as time goes on, knowledge changes and grows, and I realised that there are some useful and interesting things to be learned from considering the wider context of this and related areas. So, in this book I have expanded many of the sections to offer explanation and exploration of some of the deeper questions and issues, as well as sharing details of the more recent research and knowledge that has been published and discussed in relation to the administration of vitamin K to babies.

The book is divided into five sections. In the first, I'll take you through the different elements of the vitamin K decision. In section two we will look at the bigger picture and some of the wider questions that people ask about this topic (although I won't pretend that I have good answers to all of these). The theme of questions continues into section three, which is a 'pot pourri' of frequently asked questions, either asked or sent to me by parents and others interested in this area. Section four includes some stories from women who have written about their experiences and decision making process, and the book closes with section five, which offers a few signposts for parents who make different decisions about vitamin K.

I hope this book serves you well. I continue to look out for research and new thinking in this area and, if you would like to keep in touch with this, you may like to visit my website at www.sarawickham.com, where you can also sign up to a free monthly newsletter in which I share research and other information relating to pregnancy, birth and women's health.

Sara Wickham.
Wiltshire, England. Summer 2017.

1 Exploring the decision

Your baby, your decision

I hope you already know that the vitamin K decision, like all birth-related decisions, is yours to make as a parent. I'm not going to claim that it's always an easy decision, but it is your decision. You might decide to follow the local recommendation and have vitamin K given to your baby. You might decide to ask for oral (given by mouth) vitamin K rather than injected vitamin K or to look for another alternative. You might decide to decline vitamin K and wait and watch your baby or perhaps say you need more time to think about it. But the decision is for you and your family to make. With a couple of exceptions in places where parents' rights are restricted by law, parents have the right to accept or decline this type of treatment for their baby.

There is no universally right or wrong decision either. The best decision is the one that is right for you and your family and baby. Not what's right for your sister or friend or paediatrician or for somebody else's baby.

Our modern approach to health care has brought us many wonderful technologies and advances, but it has also brought what I would describe as a problematic degree of standardisation. That is, we've somehow ended up in a situation in which policymakers and professionals make decisions and recommendations about what is good for us on a population basis. They then develop so-called pathways dictating the health care journey that should be offered to everyone in a specific situation or with a certain condition. The administration of vitamin K is one of a number of things that are done in the hour or two after a baby is born and, because it has been part of the routine for so long, staff often simply assume that the offer of vitamin K will be accepted.

But we are all individuals, and the same path might not work for all of us. We come in different shapes, sizes and colours and we exhibit a staggeringly large degree of variation from each other. This variation isn't just physical. We also vary in other important regards such as how we respond to stress, what foods make us feel healthy, how much sleep we need and what is important to us. What's right for one woman, family or baby isn't necessarily right for another.

Large organisations such as systems of health care are difficult to manage. They tend to be organised around the idea of having standard pathways and guidelines that tell employees what to do, offer or recommend in particular circumstances. But those guidelines are usually not policies or laws, and it is up to individual users of the service to decide whether a recommendation is right for them or for their baby.

For that and many other reasons, parents may wish to consider what they want to do about vitamin K and other birth-related decisions before their baby is born. That doesn't mean that a pre-birth decision should be a hard-and-fast one, because situations change and factors and knowledge may emerge during the birth journey that might change what you would have decided to do. But too many parents face such decisions immediately after a baby's birth, when they may be tired and perhaps not be in the best state to ask questions or obtain more information. So the aim of this book is to help you understand the issues so that you can think about which path is right for you and your baby.

What is vitamin K?

Vitamin K is a fat-soluble substance, stored in the liver, that is needed for the complex process of blood clotting. It is an essential substance for the human body (which is why it is termed a vitamin, as the term derives from the Latin word for life) and the scientists who discovered it in the 1940s were awarded a Nobel Prize for their work.

The main function of vitamin K in the human body is in preventing bleeding through the formation of blood clots, although it may also be important in promoting good bone health. When a blood clot is needed by the body, small blood cells (platelets) are broken down to form a network of protein fibre called fibrin. A number of other substances that are carried in the blood then 'fill in' this network to form the clot, and vitamin K is needed for the manufacture of several of these substances.

There are two forms of naturally-occurring vitamin K: vitamin K_1 and vitamin K_2. Vitamin K_1 is found naturally in certain kinds of food, such as green leafy vegetables. It is known as the plant form of vitamin K and animals (including humans) can convert vitamin K_1 into vitamin K_2 with the help of gut bacteria. Vitamin K_2 comes in several variations but we will focus on vitamin K_1 here because the synthetic form of this is the kind of vitamin K offered to babies.

The pharmaceutical preparation also contains one or more oils in which the vitamin K is dissolved. The oil helps ensure that the vitamin K is released into the body over time, rather than all at once. This is why we call it depot administration when we give vitamin K by injection, because a depot of the drug is formed when it is dissolved in oil and injected into a muscle. This depot of the vitamin K is then released slowly into the baby's tissue over a period of several weeks.

It is very rare for an adult to be deficient in vitamin K, although this can happen when a person experiences certain diseases (e.g. liver or bowel disease) or takes some kinds of pharmaceutical drugs (e.g. anticoagulants or barbiturates). But a very small number of babies experience a rare but serious bleeding disorder. This disorder was first named haemorrhagic disease of the newborn (HDN) and has since come to be called vitamin K deficiency bleeding (VKDB). A few decades ago, Swedish doctor and researcher Jörgen Lehmann (1944) discovered that giving vitamin K to all newborn babies reduced the incidence of this disorder. Ever since, it has been the policy of most high-income countries to offer vitamin K to all newborn babies, and the majority of babies in these countries now receive vitamin K at birth.

Giving babies vitamin K is a little bit like giving a vaccine. The disease that it prevents is rare, but it can be very serious. We don't know ahead of time which babies might be affected by VKDB, so we offer the preventative measure to every baby. I want to stress, however, that vitamin K is not a vaccine. It is a routinely recommended form of prophylaxis, or preventative medical care.

As prophylaxis is such an important concept in relation to vitamin K (and, in fact, many other decisions that parents need to make throughout the childbearing and childrearing journey), I'd like to discuss what this means in more depth. Then I'll look at the questions that we should ask when deciding whether or not to have a prophylactic treatment and consider the answers to those questions in relation to vitamin K.

Pondering prophylaxis

The word prophylaxis is defined in various dictionaries as a drug, treatment or action that is taken to prevent disease. Examples of prophylactic treatment include the antibiotics that are given during a surgical procedure to prevent possible infection, the statin drugs that some people take in the hope of reducing their chance of heart disease and, as I already mentioned, vaccines. Within maternity care, other examples of prophylactic drugs include the anti-D that a rhesus negative woman might decide to have in the hope of preventing rhesus sensitisation (which can sometimes affect a future baby) and the oxytocic drugs that may be given after the baby's birth to facilitate the birth of the placenta.

Prophylaxis doesn't only come in the form of drugs or chemical substances. Putting on a seatbelt when we travel in a car or aeroplane could be considered prophylactic. In such situations, we hope that the vehicle won't be involved in an accident or a sudden stop but, on the rare occasion when that happens, the seatbelt offers a degree of protection.

Most people don't mind wearing a seatbelt in those circumstances, and there aren't too many risks or downsides to doing so. In many countries, wearing a seatbelt is also a legal requirement, so there are other consequences of not wearing one. When it comes to medical prophylaxis, it's probably fair to say that a good number of people will also decide to go along with government advice on prevention or their care provider's recommendation that they or their baby would benefit from having a particular drug or treatment. But some won't want to do that. Some people will want to look at the evidence for themselves and think more deeply about whether a drug or treatment is right for them or their baby. They might want to consider the pros and cons of prophylactic drugs, so that they can weigh up the benefits and downsides of the options that are open to them.

Over my years of practising and teaching midwifery, I have developed a tool that helps people to remember six key questions that we can ask of a prophylactic treatment in order to help decide whether it is something that we would want to take (or do) ourselves or give to our baby. Firstly, here are the questions:

1. What is the **problem**? That is, what problem are we trying to prevent, and how serious is the problem? In the case of vitamin K, the problem that we are trying to prevent is a disease called vitamin K deficiency bleeding (VKDB) and we will look at that next.

2. What is the **incidence**? A person could also ask how

likely is it that, without the prophylaxis, they or their baby will experience that particular problem. Again, there's a discussion on this below.

3. How **effective** is prophylaxis? In other words, how likely is it that the prophylactic treatment will prevent the problem? This isn't always as clear cut as we might like, but I will guide you through this question and share evidence on the effectiveness of different routes of administration.

4. What are the **downsides**? Are there risks of taking the prophylactic treatment, and how likely are they? The downsides can include side effects and wider issues. More on this below too.

5. Are there any **alternatives** to the prophylactic treatment? I will look at the alternatives that some people have considered, including the alternative approach of watchful waiting.

6. Finally, I suggest that people need to consider what is right for **you**, as an individual, and/or your baby. There are two elements of this. The first involves considering whether there are things about particular people or situations that change any of the population-level information in the other areas that we have looked at. For instance, if a drug doesn't work so well in people with blue eyes, or if the incidence of the problem is higher in a particular city. Secondly, I suggest to parents that they consider their own health history, family situation, thoughts, beliefs, feelings and ability to cope in different situations, as all of these factors and more can make a difference as to whether a decision or intervention is right in your individual circumstances.

I have put the key words in each of these sentences in

bold because I use these keywords and the acronym PIEDAY (which are the initial letters of problem, incidence, effectiveness, downsides, alternatives and you) when teaching midwifery and medical students, and I have also shared them with many parents. If you have the kind of mind that likes this way of thinking, it can be a useful way of remembering the key questions to ask of any prophylaxis or medical treatment that you are offered.

What is the problem? HDN or VKDB

Haemorrhagic disease of the newborn (HDN) was first described over a hundred years ago (Townsend 1894) as a spontaneous bleeding syndrome occasionally seen in newborn babies. Doctors realised that it was different from bleeding caused by trauma or inherited bleeding disorders like haemophilia. Now more commonly known as vitamin K deficiency bleeding (VKDB), this disorder is divided into three time frames. The causes of each are different. Confusingly, some authors of medical papers now refer to just two time frames; early and late VKDB. However, most have stuck with the original classification so I have shared the original one as it is still more common.

Early onset VKDB is very rare. This disorder occurs within 24 hours of birth and it is seen in babies born to women who are taking certain kinds of drugs, including anticonvulsants, anticoagulants (e.g. warfarin) or antibiotics (Darlow and Harding 1995, Gopakumar *et al* 2010). This disorder cannot be prevented by giving vitamin K to babies and we will not be considering it further here.

Classic onset VKDB is said to occur between the second and seventh days of a baby's life (although in the newer definitions that I mentioned above, some authors define early onset VKDB as occurring anytime from birth until two weeks of age). A baby who has classic onset VKDB may have bleeding under the skin, in the gut, from the nose or from a circumcision wound (Puckett and Offringa 2002). Vitamin K is given at birth in the hope of preventing both this and the next type (or time frame) of VKDB.

Late onset VKDB describes bleeding occurring between eight days (or two weeks according to some authors) and three months of age, although it has also been described occurring in babies of up to four months of age (Schulte *et al* 2014). In some of the babies who have late onset VKDB, this is associated with unrecognised liver disease and is not prevented by the administration of vitamin K at birth (Enkin *et al* 2002). In fact, underlying liver disease can actually be masked if vitamin K has been given at birth (see Emma's story on page 75). However, late onset bleeding can occasionally occur in babies who were not given vitamin K at birth (Schulte *et al* 2014). With this type of VKDB, the most common sites of bleeding are the skin, gut and brain (Puckett and Offringa 2002).

Babies who experience vitamin K deficiency bleeding will generally be admitted to a neonatal intensive care unit (NICU). Their parents or caregivers may spot that they have bleeding, or the condition may present with other symptoms, for instance poor feeding, fussiness, sleepiness, change in pallor (skin colour) and/or vomiting. The length of time that a baby who has been diagnosed with VKDB will need to spend in hospital will depend on the severity of bleeding, any complications and the baby's response to treatment. Babies presenting with VKDB will be given vitamin K. Other possible treatments include giving the baby blood products.

The most severe complication of VKDB is intracranial haemorrhage (ICH) (bleeding within the brain). When this occurs, surgery may sometimes be needed to relieve the pressure caused by bleeding. In a UK survey of VKDB and related issues, 30% of babies with VKDB had ICH (McNinch *et al* 2007). The outcome for a baby who has an ICH depends on the severity and location of the haemorrhage; in the McNinch *et al* (2007) survey of British paediatricians, there were a total of 66 cases of VKDB and two of the babies died.

ICH can also lead to brain damage. In a later UK study (Busfield et al 2012), none of the 11 babies who experienced VKDB died, but four had ICH and in two cases it was thought that the baby would have long-term problems. Of the seven babies described in one US case series who were thought to have VKDB, four were known to have ICH and two of these required urgent surgery. All of the babies in this case series also survived, although three of the babies were noted as having ongoing neurological problems or developmental delays; one case was described as mild, one considered moderate and one was thought to be severe (Schulte *et al* 2014).

Babies who experience VKDB but who do not have ICH and are otherwise healthy tend to have a good prognosis. They will be treated with vitamin K and they usually respond very quickly to this. As Gopakumar *et al* (2010) note, *"Except in the face of serious internal bleeding, reversal of the vitamin K deficiency by the administration of vitamin K is generally adequate. If there is no hepatic [that is, liver] dysfunction, its administration is followed by an increase in prothrombin time above the minimal level required for hemostasis within 3 to 4 h[ours], and usually a return to normal in about 24 h[ours]."*

What is the incidence of VKDB?

I am aware that my description of vitamin K deficiency bleeding in the previous section sounds pretty scary. I have absolutely no desire to scare parents (or anyone else for that matter), but it's important to understand that VKDB can be serious. If it wasn't serious and in many cases preventable, health systems wouldn't spend so much time and money offering vitamin K to all babies. But another key factor in the decision making process is how common or rare such a problem is.

It is difficult to be certain about exactly what proportion of babies would be at risk of VKDB if they did not receive vitamin K. This is mainly because we began to give vitamin K to almost all babies before we had really good methods of counting and measuring disease and the effectiveness of prophylaxis or treatment in the population as a whole. Some people (including myself) lament the fact that we do not have good data from a randomised controlled trial on late onset VKDB (Slattery 1994). Instead, we only have a couple of small trials on classic onset VKDB. In theory, a really large randomised controlled trial – where we gave half the babies vitamin K and half a placebo – could tell us more about the incidence of VKDB, the effectiveness of vitamin K and, just as importantly, the frequency and nature of any associated adverse events. But in practice, it would likely be considered unethical to carry out such a trial. That's because we have reason to believe from other kinds of studies and from our experience of giving vitamin K to babies for so many years that it is very effective. People would argue that it was unethical to deny vitamin K to the babies in the placebo group of the trial.

Early researchers in this field estimated that, before vitamin K was given routinely, around 1 in every 10,000 healthy newborn babies suffered from VKDB (McNinch and Tripp 1991, Von Kries and Hanawa 1993, Passmore *et al*

1988). Later reviews suggested that, in Europe, between 1 in 14,000 and 1 in 25,000 babies were affected by late onset VKDB without prophylaxis (Shearer 2009). More recently, Sankar *et al* (2016) conducted a systematic review of this area for the World Health Organization (WHO) in relation to global rates of late onset VKDB, and their figures show that,

> *"The median (interquartile range) burden of late VKDB was 35 (10.5 to 80) per 100 000 live births in infants who had not received prophylaxis at birth; the burden was much higher in low- and middle-income countries as compared with high-income countries - 80 (72 to 80) vs 8.8 (5.8 to 17.8) per 100 000 live births."* (Sankar *et al* 2016)

In other words, the incidence of late onset VKDB is higher in babies born in low-income and middle-income countries and much lower in high-income countries. If you are living in a high-income country, the average chance of a baby experiencing late onset VKDB without vitamin K prophylaxis is 1 in 11,363. There is some variation in this figure, depending on which study you look at, and this variation is inevitable with something that happens quite rarely. You'll also find that people round the figures up or down a bit, mainly because whole numbers are often easier to make sense of. The exact incidence in the studies that Sankar *et al* (2016) looked at ranged from 1 in 5,617 to 1 in 17,241 and some researchers, such as Lippi and Franchini (2011) have offered a slightly different figure in the shape of an estimate of the incidence in babies who do not have vitamin K but who are fully breastfed: between 1 in 15,000 and 1 in 20,000.

If all of these numbers are a bit confusing, here's what I say to parents on this question. The estimates of the incidence of late onset VKDB in babies who don't receive vitamin K are varied, and that's inevitable with this kind of research. The figure varies from 1 in 5600 to 1 in 25,000 but the average incidence of late onset VKDB in high-income countries in a robust WHO study is about 1 in 11,000, so that's the number that I tend to think about myself.

I think it is important to note that some authors have recently published estimates of the incidence of VKDB that differ wildly from those that I have just shared. I want to provide details of those and also explain why I and other people disagree with these so that you can weigh up the arguments and decide for yourself what you think. The figures are rather worrying, as they claim that up to 1 in 59 babies are affected by late onset VKDB. This is clearly a very different proposition to the figure that I've just quoted of 1 in about 11,000. Let's look at what is behind this difference.

In June 2014, an article was published in a paediatric journal (Schulte *et al* 2014). The authors shared details of four babies who experienced late onset VKDB and were admitted to one large tertiary care hospital in Tennessee, USA over an eight-month period. This and related papers (including Warren *et al* 2013 and CDC 2013) also discussed three other babies admitted to the same hospital who were suspected to have VKDB or found to have low levels of vitamin K upon laboratory testing. The paediatricians working at this hospital were understandably very concerned about this situation.

Before I look further at the Tennessee figures, I want to note something important. Because vitamin K is an effective form of prophylaxis, as we'll look at in more depth below, it is inevitable that almost all of the babies who go on to develop VKDB these days will not have received this at birth, either because their parents declined it or for another reason, for instance that it was forgotten.

Some people took the numbers from the series of cases of VKDB in Tennessee and argued that the chance of a baby experiencing VKDB is far higher than the WHO figure discussed above (Sankar *et al* 2016). The Tennessee case series being quoted on the internet and in American midwifery literature by others (e.g. Dekker 2014, Phillippi *et al* 2016) but a number of doctors, midwives and parents' rights groups are concerned that this claim is misleading and not based on sound evidence.

The main concern about the validity of this statement is that the numbers used to calculate the new alleged risk did not result from a carefully designed and controlled research study, but from a crude calculation based upon a series of events occurring in one area. There could have been factors that we do not know about which affected this situation. Another important issue is that it is not uncommon for hospitals and specialist units to sometimes experience a 'run' of a particular problem or situation. While vigilance is important when we see an apparently unusual pattern or an increase in the frequency of a situation, we need to take care to remember that we might just be seeing an anomalous series of events. Such occurrences are worth investigating, but we need to look at a much wider sample using carefully thought out research methods in order to determine whether our previous knowledge was incorrect or whether we are looking at a statistical anomaly.

A comparison could be made to the news stories which report on phenomena such as when ten of the twelve women who work in one small business become pregnant in the same year. It looks and seems incredible when it happens, but if you then discover that there are three thousand small businesses that employ twelve women just in one state and the other 2,999 didn't have this experience, an apparently significant event seems less remarkable.

Another example commonly used by statistics lecturers to illustrate the idea of apparently significant (but actually anomalous and unrepresentative) sequences involves the idea of asking 5,000 people to toss a coin ten times. With that many people in the sample, some are going to have amazing results; perhaps ten heads in a row, or an interesting pattern of heads and tails. Such an event can seem incredible and significant to that person and to those around them, but when you look at the bigger picture and the fact that the other 4,999 people got more average results, it puts it into perspective.

We need to put the Tennessee experience into perspective and consider that, as distressing as it must have been both for the parents and the clinicians involved, this was likely an anomalous sequence and not evidence of a sudden change in the incidence of VKDB. While I applaud those who spotted this trend and investigated it, because this is often how advances are made in medicine, it is important to ask whether anywhere else in the world has experienced a change that should cause us to reconsider the long-accepted figures. This could help us determine whether the Tennessee experience was a one-off anomalous event or the first sign of an increase in the incidence of VKDB.

To my knowledge, and after searching the literature and having a number of conversations with paediatricians in several countries, I have not found any other suggestion that higher than usual rates of VKDB are being seen elsewhere, even where rates of parents who decline vitamin K are similar to those cited in the papers written about the Tennessee experience.

In addition, the systematic review by Sankar *et al* (2016) was a robust study that was funded by the Department of Maternal, Newborn, Child and Adolescent Health and Development at the WHO. We can thus be confident of its validity. The risk of late onset VKDB in a healthy newborn baby born in a high-income country is between 1 in 5,617 and 1 in 17,241. This averages out at about 1 baby in 11,000.

How effective is prophylaxis?

Vitamin K prophylaxis is very effective. If the appropriate dose is given at the appropriate time and via the appropriate route, the chance of a baby experiencing VKDB goes from low (1 in 5,617 to 1 in 17,241) to extremely low (estimated as

1 in 100,000, although we don't have an exact figure).

Lehmann's 1944 study was the first research paper to be published on this topic. His team gave 1mg of oral vitamin K_3 (menadione) to 13,000 newly born babies and showed that the babies given vitamin K were less likely to die from a haemorrhage than the babies who didn't receive vitamin K. That was the first suggestion that vitamin K was effective, although we need to take care when looking at older studies such as this one, because there are a number of differences between what was happening then and what happens today.

One feature of Lehmann's (1944) study illustrates why we need to consider elements of a prophylactic intervention other than effectiveness. The first studies in this area used a different kind of vitamin K than is given today. Lehmann's (1944) study used a synthetic form of vitamin K called vitamin K_3. However, this form of vitamin K was found to damage blood cells and some of the babies experienced brain damage as a result of unresolved jaundice (Sankar *et al* 2016). When scientists learned how to make a synthetic version of vitamin K_1, this was used instead. (We'll turn to the question of side effects of vitamin K_1 next).

There have not been any scientific trials evaluating the effectiveness of vitamin K in relation to late onset VKDB, but two randomised trials have evaluated the effect of giving an injection of vitamin K into a muscle (also known as intramuscular or IM vitamin K) on the risk of classic onset VKDB, which occurs between the second and seventh days of a baby's life. First, Vietti *et al* (1960) gave 5mg of vitamin K_1 to baby boys who were born on even-numbered days (which was an early example of how researchers would randomly allocate babies to different groups) and who were going to undergo circumcision. The babies who had vitamin K were far less likely to bleed after circumcision than the babies who did not have vitamin K. It is important to bear in mind when we consider the results of this study that most babies do not experience circumcision or another surgical intervention that can cause bleeding.

A few years later, Sutherland *et al* (1967) compared two different dosages of vitamin K₃ with a placebo. They found that vitamin K reduced both the incidence and severity of bleeding. Both of these studies have been used to illustrate the claim that there are poor levels of vitamin K in breast milk, yet an important caveat is that both were carried out at a time when women were (wrongly) being taught and told to breastfeed in a regimented and somewhat unnatural manner. New mothers were told, for instance, to limit their baby to a certain number of minutes on each breast and to 'artificially' time feeds rather than responding to their baby's needs. In some areas, babies were starved for the first two or three days after birth, which would have depleted their vitamin K stores. So we cannot know from these studies whether the results would have been different if women had been able to breastfeed in a less restricted, more instinctive, baby-led way.

The effectiveness of intramuscular vitamin K is also – almost coincidentally – confirmed by results of the studies that have compared this to oral vitamin K. Although no intervention can offer protection to one hundred per cent of those who receive it, the failure rate of IM vitamin K prophylaxis is estimated at 1 in 100,000, so we can be confident that IM vitamin K is very effective.

The question of effectiveness in oral vitamin K is a more complex one. Although the very first researchers looking at this area gave vitamin K orally, we have long known that oral vitamin K isn't as effective as IM vitamin K. Some health systems have always offered oral vitamin K, however, partly because it is more palatable (no pun intended) for some parents. In fact, vitamin K is a very bitter substance and is actually quite *un*palatable, which may be why some babies try to spit it out when they are given it orally.

Over the years, discussions in medical circles have focused on finding the right dosage and frequency of administration to ensure that babies receive ongoing protection when they have oral vitamin K (von Kries 1999). The biggest concern is that protection should last long enough to prevent late onset VKDB. Remember that, when vitamin K is injected into a baby's muscle, a depot of the drug is formed in the baby's tissue, so the vitamin is released into the baby's body over several weeks.

A number of research studies have been carried out over the past couple of decades, and we do now seem to have some agreement about what constitutes effective oral prophylaxis. Researchers agree that this needs to be multi-dose (Busfield *et al* 2007, Shearer 2009, van Winckel *et al* 2009, Laubscher *et al* 2013) and that the dosage and frequency need to be higher than was the case in the early regimens. A single oral dose at birth gives some protection against earlier bleeding, but up to 1 in 15,625 babies will still experience late onset VKDB (Busfield *et al* 2007). However, a Danish study revealed no cases of VKDB amongst about 396,000 babies who received weekly oral prophylaxis of 1mg of vitamin K per week from birth until three months of age (Hansen *et al* 2003).

In contrast, a Dutch study carried out a few years later (Ijland *et al* 2008) evaluated the practice of giving breastfed babies 1mg of vitamin K orally at birth, followed by a daily dose of 25 micrograms of vitamin K from 1 to 13 weeks of age. The researchers in this team found that this reduced VKDB but didn't eradicate it. This may be explained by Lippi and Franchini's (2011) observation that up to 70 per cent of the vitamin K given to babies orally is excreted in their bile and urine within a few days.

Parents who are considering oral vitamin K may be heartened to know that the Danish dosage regime seems to be effective. Unfortunately, the formulation of vitamin K that was tested in the Danish research (called Konakion or Cremophor) is no longer given to babies (Shearer 2009). Its replacement (Konakion MM) has been found to be less effective in babies with liver disease (or cholestasis), who cannot properly absorb the drug (Shearer 2009).

Clarke and Shearer (2007) distinguish the two doses used in the above studies, describing the lower Dutch dose as physiological and the Danish dose as pharmaceutical. They further note, especially in relation to the lower dose, that the absorption of vitamin K is greatly enhanced by the presence of other fats. In fact, Shearer (2009) later addresses this in more depth, explaining that, *"it cannot be assumed that a 50 µg drop preparation [or oral vitamin K] given in isolation, often on an empty stomach, would be as well absorbed as the same dose contained in a formula feed. Being fat-soluble, the absorption of VK is likely to be very poor unless taken with a feed that has bile-salt stimulating properties"*. So parents choosing oral vitamin K need to know that this isn't likely to be absorbed unless it is given with breast milk or an alternative.

Both Clarke and Shearer (2007) and McNinch *et al* (2007) note the increased effectiveness of the oral regimes offered in the UK in the past few years, while also discussing the issue of compliance. They suggest that non-compliance with giving repeated doses of oral vitamin K regimes may be even more problematic if not for the fact that many of the parents who decide to give their babies oral vitamin K are motivated, breastfeeding and perhaps more inclined than average to ensure they give the appropriate dosage at the appropriate times. This is further supported by the findings of the Swiss Paediatric Surveillance Unit (Laubscher *et al* 2013), which monitored the incidence of VKDB from July 2005 until June 2011. They found that, compared with historical controls who had received two oral doses of vitamin K, the incidence of VKDB was significantly lower in babies who had received three oral doses.

In conclusion, we can see that vitamin K is very effective as a prophylactic treatment against the chance of a baby experiencing VKDB. Intramuscular vitamin K is almost a hundred per cent effective and, although oral vitamin K is not quite as effective unless it is given repeatedly and in significant doses, there do exist oral regimens that confer a reasonable level of protection for parents who would prefer to give their babies vitamin K by this route. Oral vitamin K should always be given with a feed in order to increase the likelihood that it will be properly absorbed. The effectiveness of oral vitamin K is strongly related to dose, preparation and parents' or caregivers' ability to give this to their baby at the right times and in the right volume to give their baby ongoing protection.

What are the downsides to prophylaxis?

So VKDB is a rare but serious disease and vitamin K is very effective at preventing it, which means the next question to consider is whether there are the risks and/or downsides to giving vitamin K. As for any drug, problems might arise because of the drug itself, or as a side effect of the excipients, which are the substances that are added to the drug, such as preservatives or vehicles for carrying the drug, or as a consequence of the way that it is given.

For instance, there are a few risks that exist with any injection. One is the possibility that the injection will result in local infection, bleeding, bruising or pain at the injection site. This is uncommon and, although it may be uncomfortable, it is usually short-lived. It can be relieved by breastfeeding or cuddling the baby and doesn't usually cause other ill-effects. More seriously but also very rarely, a baby may be given the wrong drug. Drug errors have occurred when Syntometrine or pethidine (which are both used in maternity care, but intended for women rather than babies) have been given instead of vitamin K (Whitfield and Salfield 1980). Such errors can have grave consequences, but this is a risk that concerned parents can potentially reduce themselves, by asking that the vitamin K be given only in their presence. Many practitioners will do this in any case, and safety protocols are in place in the hope of preventing errors. There has been at least one case of a baby experiencing anaphylactic shock after the administration of vitamin K (Koklu *et al* 2014), but this is incredibly rare.

When it comes to considering excipients, we face a few challenges. One is that it's hard to separate out the effect of a drug and the effect of an excipient (or a combination of excipients), and this is compounded by the fact that different pharmaceutical companies will use different excipients and these also change over time as we learn more. When you look up some of the ingredients that are used in injectable versions of vitamin K, they sound awful. The version of vitamin K used in the UK, for example, contains sodium hydroxide (otherwise known as caustic soda, and a common ingredient in drain cleaner) and hydrochloric acid, which many people know to be a corrosive substance. Yet both are used in miniscule quantities in vitamin K, both are licensed and considered safe for food and drug use and both are commonly eaten or used in food production. Hydrochloric acid is found in the human stomach, where it plays a vital role in digestion, and it is used in the production of many foods. Sodium hydroxide has many food-related uses, with one of the more interesting being that it is sprayed on pretzels to make them chewy.

The UK version of vitamin K also contains glycocholic acid, which is used as an emulsifier in vitamin K injections, but is also used as a pharmaceutical treatment in its own right. In this context, it has been argued to be safe in children (Heubi *et al* 2014), although some countries' formulations of vitamin K contain emulsifiers that have not been tested or which have been the cause of question or concern. These emulsifiers may be made from animal products.

The UK vitamin K preparation is one of those that contains lecithin; a generic term for substances derived from plants or animals that help smooth the texture of oils. Lecithin is found in many foods and is not considered harmful. In fact, many excipients sound much less harmful when one knows what they are and where else they exist, but that doesn't mean that all excipients used in drugs are safe. Parents who are concerned about this can ask to see the product information of the formulation of vitamin K that is being offered in their area.

The UK and some other countries have set up surveillance systems to monitor drug effectiveness and adverse reactions. These structures work better in some countries than others, but in theory they are designed to help improve the safety of pharmaceutical drugs and ensure that these products are as safe as possible. But not everybody will be reassured by the fact that these substances are approved and monitored by regulatory bodies. In my experience, one of the concerns that the few parents who decline vitamin K have is that they don't want to have any foreign substances injected into their baby, even in miniscule quantities. Karen, a new mother in the US, wrote that, *I know it's only salt and vinegar, but that doesn't reassure me. I don't want to have salt and vinegar injected into my baby*".

Other parents are concerned that the concentration of vitamin K in a baby's body after IM administration of 1mg of vitamin K is thousands of times that of naturally occurring (endogenous) vitamin K. We do not know what effect, if any, this has on the baby other than that, as above, it provides protection against a bleed. In fact, premature babies in some areas are given less vitamin K than is given to babies born at full term. This is because of concerns about the volume that remains in their system (Lippi and Franchini 2011). Costakos *et al* (2003) showed that preterm babies who were given 0.5 to 1mg of vitamin K had vitamin K levels that were 1900 to 2600 times higher than normal adult plasma values two days after administration and 550 to 600 times higher than normal adult plasma values ten days after administration.

The final and most complex question that we need to consider here is the safety of vitamin K itself, although safety concerns have mainly been limited to the injectable form of vitamin K. In fact, the oral administration of vitamin K began or continued in some areas because of these safety concerns. Unfortunately, the question of the safety of vitamin K isn't easy to answer. There is a lack of adequately-sized research trials that could give us a sense of the actual risks by showing us the comparative outcomes in large numbers of babies who did or did not have vitamin K (Slattery 1994). As with so many areas of maternity and medical care, when something becomes common practice, it is difficult or impossible to carry out research that deprives some people of the intervention and gives them a placebo.

There are two more elements of this area that are equally unfortunate. One is that, back in the 1990s, the British press caused a big scare about the potential risks of vitamin K after the publication of a piece of research by Golding *et al* (1992) in the British Medical Journal. I'll explain this and the attending evidence further below. The second problem is that several health services and professionals haven't properly acknowledged and responded to parents' understandable concerns. Instead, they have promoted ideas that parents know (or later find out) to be untrue (including that vitamin K carries no risk at all and that the likelihood of VKDB is vastly higher than it is) and some have taken a patriarchal, heavy-handed approach towards parents' decision making about vitamin K. I will consider this later in the book, but I mention it here because I think it is important for us all to consider not just what information is available, but how it is presented. It's relatively easy to scare women and families into making a decision by emphasising risk and giving 'fear-based' information. It's harder to strike a balance where one is honest without being unnecessarily scary and to take a compassionate and gentle approach to communicating information without glossing over the enormity of some of the possible outcomes.

The most honest thing that I can say about the potential downsides of giving vitamin K to a baby is that, while we are confident that it does more good than harm on a population basis, we don't have enough data to be certain of what the possible side effects might be and how many babies they affect. We have concerns, speculation and a whole load of pages on the internet where people who don't really understand the issues share their thoughts (or their interpretation of others' thoughts), but very little real data.

I think we can say with a degree of confidence that, if vitamin K caused a really serious and unusual outcome, we would likely have spotted that by now, as the example of thalidomide showed. But there has been lots of controversy about whether IM vitamin K might increase a baby's chance of having childhood cancer, so let me spell out the history of this controversy.

In 1992, a paper was published in the British Medical Journal (Golding *et al* 1992). The authors of this study stated that its aim was, *"…to assess unexpected associations between childhood cancer and pethidine given in labour and the neonatal administration of vitamin K that had emerged in a study performed in the 1970 national birth cohort."* Golding *et al* (1992) reported on a case-control study carried out in two hospitals in Bristol, England. Their results showed that the incidence of cancer in children who had received vitamin K at birth was twice that of children who had received either no vitamin K or an oral dose only. They also wrote that a link between IM vitamin K and childhood cancer was *"biologically plausible"*. Their paper was picked up by the press, leading to a media outcry and a sizeable number of parents declining IM vitamin K. This series of events was unfortunate because, as with the Tennessee data described earlier in the book, this was a small group of babies and the information was observational rather than the result of a large, robust study.

What happened afterwards was also unfortunate, and here we have to return to the question of professional honesty. After the publication of the Golding *et al* (1992) paper, a number of researchers and clinicians rushed to try to correct and clarify what was being reported. But this is almost always easier said than done. Inaccuracy of reporting medical research sadly continues today, and irresponsible journalism is rife. Medical journals contain a stream of correspondence and writing on this issue. Some authors and clinicians have misunderstood or misrepresented what happened, and tell parents that the Golding *et al* (1992) study was refuted and thus there is no chance that IM vitamin K causes childhood cancer. This is a logical fallacy. The Golding study was undertaken because data had shown a higher rate of childhood cancer in babies who had IM vitamin K, so the discrediting of that study didn't mean that the possible association disappeared. It meant that we needed to go back to the drawing board and design a larger and better study to investigate this concern.

Most of the studies published in the aftermath of the Golding study did not find an association between childhood cancer and vitamin K (for example, Ansell *et al* 1996, McKinney *et al* 1998, Roman *et al* 2002). There are some differences of opinion about whether those studies were well-designed enough to rule out the possible link altogether. Some people conclude that, because the link has not been confirmed, we should reassure parents that it doesn't exist. Clarke and Shearer noted in 2007 that no convincing evidence had emerged in the last 15 years to support the cancer link, particularly with respect to providing any biochemical plausibility for the alleged carcinogenicity of vitamin K_1, and they also note that the preparations used today are known to have safer excipients, which I have discussed above.

Other people have continued to believe that, although it is important to tell parents that we cannot find a definitive link and more studies suggest the two are not linked than find an association, we are still in need of better research. Researchers have long argued that the possibility of an association between IM vitamin K and leukaemia still cannot be ruled out (Parker *et al* 1998, von Kries 1998, Roman *et al* 2002). Sankar *et al*'s (2016) systematic review noted that, *"Although later studies did not confirm the association between IM vitamin K prophylaxis and the risk of childhood cancer, the theoretical possibility of mutagenicity cannot be excluded."*

One final thought that I would like to add on this subject relates to the actual incidence of leukaemia. According to Cancer Research UK (2017), the incidence of childhood leukaemia in babies and children under the age of four in the UK is 8 per 100,000 boys and 7 per 100,000 girls. That works out at being 1 in 33,333. The worst-case possibility from the most poorly-conducted research suggested that vitamin K might double that risk, though please remember that this is a theoretical discussion only. So vitamin K might, at the most extreme estimate (which is almost certainly too high, and a link may not exist at all) be linked with one case of leukaemia in 16,666 children. That is still lower than our best estimate of the number of children who would have VKDB without vitamin K. This is also the conclusion drawn by Lippi and Franchini (2011): *"Although it might be concluded that there is no definitive evidence, the confirmed benefits of vitamin K prophylaxis seem to largely outweigh the hypothetical association with childhood cancer."*

It is one thing to comment on what is best on a population level, however, and quite another to consider what might be best for an individual baby, woman or family. Parents who are concerned about either any vitamin K or vitamin K by the intramuscular route have long been asking questions about what the alternative options are, so that is the question that we will consider next.

The range of alternatives

Although it might seem as if parents have a binary decision to make here – that is, give vitamin K or do not give vitamin K – there are actually a range of actions that parents can take, and these include:

- Decide to give IM vitamin K
- Decide to give oral vitamin K

- Decide to give IM or oral vitamin K but in a different time frame from what is usual
- Decline vitamin K but seek/try alternative measures to increase baby's vitamin K levels
- Decline vitamin K but become informed about VKDB and know what to watch for and what to do if worried
- Decline vitamin K and do nothing else.

Parents who aren't sure about whether they want to have vitamin K given to their baby often ask whether there are alternatives to this. A common question is whether it is possible for a woman to increase her baby's vitamin K levels, either in pregnancy or through breastfeeding, by increasing the amount of vitamin K in her diet or taking supplemental vitamin K. This is a logical question for, as Lippi and Franchini (2011) write, we know that vitamin K *is acquired through the diet and is prevalently present in leafy green vegetables such as spinach, Swiss chard, Brassica (e.g. cabbage, kale, cauliflower, turnip, and Brussels sprout), some fruits such as avocado, banana and kiwi, as well as in some vegetable oils, especially soybean oil. Interestingly, cooking does not remove significant amounts of vitamin K from these foods.*

However, vitamin K doesn't seem to cross the placenta very well at all, so increasing vitamin K intake during pregnancy isn't likely to make any difference to a baby. In one small study by Shearer *et al* (1982), researchers measured vitamin K levels in nine healthy pregnant women and compared their levels to the level of vitamin K found in their babies' blood. They could not detect vitamin K in each baby's cord blood. When they then gave six other pregnant women 1mg of vitamin K injected directly into their blood just before they gave birth, they could detect small amounts of vitamin K in blood taken from their babies' cords, but the levels were very low. These researchers speculated that either vitamin K doesn't cross the placenta easily, or that babies' blood doesn't contain the right substances to process the vitamin K. This is one of the findings that has caused some people to speculate that babies may be born with relatively low levels of vitamin K for good reason, as I will discuss further later.

However, taking vitamin K supplements while breastfeeding may have some value for parents who do not want to give vitamin K directly to their baby. It is a long-held view within the medical literature that breast milk contains low levels of vitamin K (Lippi and Francini 2011), although some of the research cited to support the claim that breast milk contains 'low' levels of vitamin K (a term that always begs the question of exactly what breast milk is being compared to as a standard) was carried out at a time when women were not being supported to breastfeed in ways that are now considered optimal. More recent research by Greer (2004) demonstrated that vitamin K levels in breast milk were about twice as high as the early studies had suggested.

A Japanese study (Kojima *et al* 2004) found that the concentration of vitamin K in breast milk varied according to the diet of the women concerned, but the few studies that have looked at supplementation in women have focused on supplementing with vitamin K tablets. For that reason, we don't know whether increasing a breastfeeding woman's dietary vitamin K would make a difference to her baby's chance of having VKDB, but we do know a bit more about supplementation, so I will share that before returning to the question of dietary vitamin K.

A few studies have looked at whether maternal supplementation with vitamin K increases the level of vitamin K found in breast milk. Two small studies showed that when lactating women took 5mg of vitamin K per day, the vitamin K level in their breast milk became high enough to confer what the researchers considered to be an adequate level of protection to their babies (Greer *et al* 1997, Bolisetty *et al* 1998). Although in many studies the dose of a drug ends up being arbitrarily chosen, Greer *et al*'s (1997) study helpfully confirmed that a daily 5mg vitamin K supplement led to women having twice as much vitamin K in their breast milk than if they took 2.5mg of vitamin K a day.

The same researchers found that when women took a daily 5mg vitamin K supplement, their babies had six to ten times the amount of vitamin K in their blood compared to the babies of women who didn't take a supplement. All of the babies in this study received a vitamin K injection at birth as well. This was because the study was just about seeing whether maternal supplementation would increase the breast milk vitamin K content; it was deemed unethical not to offer vitamin K as usual.

Another much larger study (Nishiguchi *et al* 1996) found that, when women took 15mg of vitamin K a day, 99.9% of their babies maintained what the researchers deemed adequate levels of vitamin K. These babies also received vitamin K themselves, though. In this case, they were given two doses of oral vitamin K within the first week after birth.

I have not been able to find any research that has looked at the relationship between maternal vitamin K supplementation and the chance of a baby having VKDB. So we have no evidence of the effectiveness of maternal vitamin K supplementation in that regard, and neither do we have data on whether there are downsides to giving a baby relatively high amounts of vitamin K in breast milk. But if a woman does not want to have vitamin K given to her baby directly, then breastfeeding and taking a supplement is an alternative she might want to consider. Some women decide to increase their dietary intake of vitamin K rather than taking a supplement. They may or may not aim to ingest 5mg of vitamin K per day but, for illustrative purposes only, 5mg of vitamin K is the amount found in five cups of cooked kale, which contains the highest known proportion of vitamin K in commonly eaten foods.

If women do wish to increase their dietary vitamin K or take supplements with the aim of giving vitamin K to their baby via breast milk, then they should be informed that there are substances that inhibit the absorption of vitamin K, including mineral oil, antibiotics, phenobarbital and phenytoin (which are sedative drugs used to treat epilepsy), anticoagulants, oral contraceptives and high doses of vitamin A. There is no direct evidence to suggest that avoiding these will make a difference, but that is because this has not been investigated.

The knowledge that supplementation and breastfeeding may be at least partially protective against VKDB begs another important question. Artificial milk has long been supplemented with vitamin K. Somewhat ironically, this supplementation may have added fuel to the idea that the levels in breast milk are 'too low'. We might then ask why, if artificial milk contains high levels of vitamin K, is vitamin K still given to babies who will be fed this?

Shearer (2009) notes that almost all cases of VKDB occur in babies who are exclusively breastfed, which would imply that artificial baby milk is also at least somewhat protective against VKDB. But I have never seen a paper or met a paediatrician who felt that feeding artificial milk was enough. I imagine a key concern is that although babies who are fed artificial milk may have lower rates of VKDB, this doesn't eradicate the condition completely. Many parents feed a combination of mother's milk and artificial milk, which would mean it was impossible to see or predict how much vitamin K a baby was receiving. There may also be a related desire not to promote artificial milk given that mother's milk confers a multitude of other advantages on both the baby and their mother.

Other parents decline vitamin K and decide to either do nothing or to wait and watch. A very few parents wait to see whether there is a reason that their particular baby might be at higher risk of VKDB. A small number of parents delay the administration of vitamin K, as I will discuss later. The parents who wait watchfully will, ideally, be aware that the baby does have a small chance of VKDB and understand what the symptoms of this look like. They will know that they need to have a low threshold for responding to any symptoms, concerns or to any breastfeeding difficulties, which are thought to increase the chance of a problem. We have no evidence about whether any of these things can make a difference. That is, again, because they haven't been researched, which is unsurprising given the medical view that vitamin K prophylaxis at birth is the best option. More on this in the final section of the book.

What's right for you and your baby?

Already it can be seen just how complex this issue is and, as is the case with many health-related decisions, there exists a fundamental tension. That is, we can only gather statistics and facts like those that I have been sharing if we look at large numbers of people, and yet parents make decisions for just one individual baby.

On the one hand, giving vitamin K to all babies on a population basis prevents most occurrences of VKDB, which is a serious condition, so this is why policymakers recommend it. On the other hand, the statistical chance of any one baby having VKDB is very small (about 1 in 11,000) and some parents are concerned about possible downsides.

It is understandable that not everybody wants to take the population-level recommendation without at least thinking about the issue for themselves. We live in a culture where the advantages of such prophylactic treatments are often promoted without much discussion of the possible associated downsides or disadvantages. But we also need to remember the enormity of the problem that vitamin K is offered to prevent. Even if only one in 11,000 babies develops a condition, if your baby is that one baby, that is one hundred percent of your and your baby's experience.

If it was possible to know which babies were going to have VKDB, the decision would become much easier. Even if parents could know that their baby was at a much lower or much higher risk of VKDB than average, then it might be easier to decide whether or not to give vitamin K. But we have very little knowledge about which babies are at risk of VKDB.

Some years ago, it was thought that it might be possible to put babies into 'low risk' and 'high risk' categories and thus offer what is known as targeted prophylaxis. This means that prophylactic vitamin K would be offered to babies who are at higher risk and not to babies who are lower risk. Sutor (2003) was among those who acknowledged the need to *"search for methods of identifying early the few infants destined to bleed so that targeted prophylaxis can replace the current 'prophylaxis for all'"*. I worked with several paediatricians who carried out work looking at this possibility, and some of the questions that were considered included whether a 'traumatic' birth (which included an instrumental birth) led to babies being at higher risk of VKDB. However, no evidence was ever found to support this theory. Sadly, very little has been published on this subject, in part because people don't tend to publish the results of research that doesn't find anything conclusive. We know for sure that some of the babies who develop VKDB have 'gentle births', sometimes at home or in birth centres (Brousseau *et al* 2005, Darlow *et al* 2011, Khambalia *et al* 2012, Schulte *et al* 2014).

So we do not have evidence that there is a link between the type of birth and the chance of a baby having VKDB. Furthermore, we know that having a gentle birth does not give a guarantee that a baby is risk-free. Discussions continue about whether certain medicalised birth practices such as early umbilical cord clamping may make a difference (for example, see Cranford 2011), but we have no evidence about this either.

A couple of other things are generally accepted in this area. Circumcision of male infants is considered to be a risk factor for VKDB. Also, many of the people who perform tongue-tie division surgery won't carry this out on babies under 12 weeks unless the baby has either received IM vitamin K or it can be demonstrated via a blood test that the baby has an adequate blood clotting result.

Paediatrician Edmund Hey (2003a) offered a really useful summary of the risk factors for VKDB when he wrote:

> *"Babies who do not feed soon, well and regularly are at measurable risk of bleeding once their limited reserves of vitamin K are exhausted. All babies who are not well enough to be fed at birth need a supplement because their vitamin K stores will only last 1-3 days.*
>
> *A few breastfed babies will develop transient VKDB if they are not given a small supplement at birth, probably because early intake is poor.*
>
> *A very small number of breastfed babies risk a sudden serious bleed when 2-12 weeks old if not offered a regular supplement, usually because an unrecognised liver disorder has impaired fat-soluble vitamin absorption."* (Hey 2003a:12)

Unfortunately, there is a limit to what we can do to identify these babies ahead of time, which is why the practice is to offer universal prophylaxis. However, this doesn't mean that we shouldn't make parents who decline vitamin K aware of possible early warning signs, and I will look at this in more depth in the final section of the book.

While these are the factors that have been considered within the midwifery and medical literature, there will also be personal factors and circumstances that individual parents will want to consider when making their decision. This individual weighing up of the issues is the final element of the PIEDAY approach (see page 9) to considering a prophylactic treatment. So, to summarise, I have looked at the problem and incidence of VKDB, the effectiveness of prophylaxis, the possible downsides, the possible alternatives and posed the all-important question of 'what's right for your baby?'. In the next section, I will go on to look at the wider issues relating to this area but I'd like to offer one final discussion before we move on, and that concerns the different forms of vitamin K that are used around the world.

Preparations, dosage and international variation

We have not yet, for the most part, considered the different preparations of vitamin K that are available, although I have mentioned a few of these (such as Konakion and Konakion MM) in relation to specific research findings. That is partly because there is a lot of variation and change in this area. Policies and products are largely dictated by what vitamin K manufacturers have decided to develop, license and market rather than by an informed understanding of what babies need (Hey 2003b). We have gaps in our knowledge about the comparative effectiveness and safety of different products, alongside vast international, national and local differences in the recommended dosage, route and frequency of administration (Sutor 2003, Tandoi *et al* 2005, Harvey 2008, van Winckel *et al* 2009, Clarke 2010, Greer 2010).

Surveys of what is happening in practice have also consistently continued to show variation. Ansell *et al* (2004) surveyed paediatricians in 20 large maternity units in the UK and reported that there had been frequent policy changes between 1977 and 2002. Busfield *et al* (2007) carried out a related study, looking firstly at the current use of vitamin K prophylaxis in the UK and then relating this to the effectiveness of the regimens used. Their research revealed wide variation in the form of vitamin K offered where babies had been born at term following uncomplicated births, with 60% recommending intramuscular prophylaxis, 24% oral vitamin K prophylaxis and 16% offering parents a choice of either route. All of the units who offered IM vitamin K in this study gave a single dose, usually 1mg of Konakion

Neonatal, and there is now consensus in the UK that this is the appropriate drug and dose for IM administration.

There continues to be considerable variation in the timing, dosage and frequency of the oral regimens that are offered (Busfield *et al* 2007) and a straw poll amongst colleagues from around the world conducted as this book was being written revealed that this situation continues, with frequent changes taking place. Guala *et al* (2005) also found wide variability in procedures between different nurseries in Italy and, in New Zealand, Robertshawe's (2009) audit unearthed variations in the way that vitamin K was prescribed and its administration documented.

Some countries do not have a vitamin K preparation that is licensed for oral use, so parents may find that this option is not open to them or that they must source it from elsewhere. According to women and practitioners that I have talked to in these areas, it is common for parents to use the internet to purchase vitamin K for oral use, as local practitioners are unable or unwilling to support or source this. Other studies highlight the continuing problem of VKDB in countries where parents also do not get to make a choice, but this time because prophylaxis is either not available or is too expensive (Danielsson *et al* 2004).

When I was writing this book, I invited questions from colleagues and parents. One of the most interesting was sent to me by Paul:

> *I wonder how much injections like vitamin K being routinely recommended for all, alongside the increase in vaccinations generally is more about making money for drug companies than for the health of our babies? How much profit do drugs companies make out of vitamin K production? Also, if it's a lot, how can those manufacturers - who are known to have strong financial links to the health-policy making governments be open to being objective about the evidence?*

I don't have good answers to Paul's questions, although in the UK a dose of Konakion Neonatal costs about 38 pence. So although he is right to point out that there is a lot of profit to be made from pharmaceutical drugs, vitamin K is comparatively inexpensive. But Paul's question illustrates that there are wider issues to be considered here, and it is those which we will look at in the next section.

2 The bigger questions

Deciding whether to give vitamin K is straightforward and easy for some people, but not for others. Many people believe that the severity of VKDB alone should warrant universal vitamin K prophylaxis. But not everyone wants their baby to be given substantial amounts of any substance that may – as we will discuss in this section of the book - alter a physiologically beneficial state, especially in the absence of good evidence about the potential downsides of giving this substance. There is concern from some quarters that some parents are making their decision based on inaccurate information, and this is almost certainly the case, as there are plenty of sources of inaccurate and/or incomplete information out there. Yet I have cared for a number of midwives, doctors and scientists who have declined vitamin K for their babies, and no-one could suggest that these parents lacked access to medical opinion and relevant literature.

Thus the issues are more complex than we might at first realise, and there are some controversies in this area that are not easily reconciled. In this part of the book, I will look more closely at some of those debates and try to answer some of the questions that people ask. Unfortunately, as we saw earlier in the book, we don't always have enough knowledge to be able to offer good answers. Even when this is the case, though, it can still be helpful to understand more about the background of the issue, the different approaches that people take towards it and what we do and don't know.

Are babies born with a vitamin K deficiency?

As you may have spotted from some of the quotes in the early part of this book (and, in fact, the very first line I wrote about what I was taught to say to parents as a student midwife), the mainstream medical viewpoint on this area has tended to be that babies are born with a vitamin K deficiency. For instance, Zipursky (1996) states, *"that all newborn infants are deficient in vitamin K is apparent from their low plasma concentrations of vitamin K and a deficiency of the vitamin K dependent coagulation factors II, VII, IX, and X"*. Even the most recent Cochrane document on this topic begins with the statement that, *"Newborn infants are deficient in vitamin K"* (Ardell *et al* 2010).

But this viewpoint has been questioned by many people (including myself) on several grounds. First, many people find it hard to believe that all babies are born without something they really need. It makes sense, such people might say, that a few babies will have problems, but would they *all* be deficient in a vital substance? Surely we would by now have evolved to have babies born rich in vitamin K if they really needed it? Maybe most babies don't need vitamin K in utero or for their first weeks of life, and maybe there is even good reason for this?

The word 'deficiency' is quite loaded. It suggests that people lack something that they need and the use of the term deficiency in relation to all babies – as opposed to its use in relation only to the tiny number of babies who do not adequately increase their vitamin K stores and go on to have a clotting problem – is a bone of contention in some areas. In fact, I wrote an article about this, many years ago, in which I raised and discussed these questions in the midwifery literature. The article was called, *'Vitamin K: a flaw in the blueprint'* and I wrote that:

"Some fairly obvious questions are raised by this statement [that all babies are deficient in vitamin K]:

· *What is a 'low' level of vitamin K?*
· *Semantically, can all babies have low levels?*
· *Low in relation to what?*
· *How do we define low levels and normal levels?*
· *Surely someone needs to have a normal level against which this is measured?*
· *Who has normal levels of vitamin K?*

Actually, although the 'all babies have a low level' argument is heard in practice and not something which I have ever seen analysed 'in the literature', babies are deemed to have low levels of vitamin K relative to adult levels. Babies also have large heads relative to adult head size, but this is not perceived as pathological. It is deemed a good thing, because the human brain needs to be large at birth. Yet the fact that relative vitamin K levels differ between newborn and adult is perceived as pathological. Why? Philosophically, the question is raised that, if all babies have what is perceived as a 'low' level of vitamin K, then surely this must become the 'normal level' of vitamin K for babies to have. Even if proponents of vitamin K think that this is 'too low' a level for some reason, they need to state this, rather than telling women their baby is deficient in an essential substance. Doesn't this just feed back into the idea that women are relatively inefficient at making babies and need to be supplemented by the skills and technology of hospitals and doctors?" (Wickham 2000)

The best thing about writing this article was that people responded to it, in a variety of ways, which meant that a dialogue could happen. Several of the responses received were from midwives and parents who said things along the lines of, *'yes, that's what I think too ... we should think more about this'.* We also received a couple of negative responses from doctors who clearly felt that I shouldn't be 'allowed' to ask such questions and challenge their authority, but the best response (at least in my view) came from a paediatrician, Edmund Hey. You might recall Edmund's name from the first section of the book, as it was he who first (to the best of my knowledge) clarified his view of the situation in the literature.

No, he suggested, nature is not flawed. But the margin of safety is narrow (Hey 2003a).

This was very helpful, because it acknowledged that most babies do have the means to build up their vitamin K to a level that will be protective for them (at least for the approximately 10,999 out of 11,000 babies who aren't affected by VKDB), but the occasional baby won't do this for one reason or another. We can't necessarily predict who that baby will be, which is why prophylaxis is offered universally, and the notion of a margin of safety now gives us a new lens through which to consider this issue.

Hey's (2003a) article did two other things. By being open to discussing the terminology used in this area, he gave us another illustration of the importance of being careful about the language that we use. His work underlined how vital it is to consider the nuances of what we are saying. There is a stark difference for some people between hearing that all babies are deficient in vitamin K (and thus switching off from even considering giving vitamin K because this statement flies in the face of their existing belief that nature works well most of the time) and being given a more nuanced explanation. His more nuanced version acknowledged that no, nature hasn't got it wrong but, for reasons we don't fully understand, there is a low margin of safety in this area. When we use the second way of talking about the issues, we are no longer implicitly questioning women, babies and the birth process by telling parents that their baby is lacking in something. This is important, because such a stance can feel patronising and off-putting to some people.

Unfortunately, Hey's work has not significantly changed what is said to parents in some areas.

Do babies have relatively low vitamin K levels for a reason?

It's possible, but we don't know. What we do know is that there seem to be a number of means through which nature (if we can use that rather tenuous concept just for the sake of discussion) has ensured that babies are receiving lower levels of vitamin K relative to adult levels. For instance: *"Infants are at higher risk for hemorrhagic disease of newborn, caused by a lack of vitamin K reaching the fetus across the placenta, the low level of vitamin K levels in breast milk, immature liver and low colonic bacterial synthesis."* (Gopakumar *et al* 2010). Medical researchers use this evidence to explain how and why there is a narrow margin of safety in this area and justify their desire to give vitamin K to all babies. Yet others use the same evidence to argue that perhaps the multiple means by which babies are prevented from receiving high volumes of vitamin K may imply that babies do not benefit from large volumes of vitamin K at this stage of their lives.

It is almost inevitable that, once people have questioned the statement that all babies are deficient in vitamin K, they go on to wonder whether there is a rationale or reason behind the fact that all babies are born with lower levels of vitamin K than older babies or adults. There are two elements of human knowledge that are important to consider when we ponder such a question. The first is that, although such questions are fascinating and tantalising, they are also almost impossible to answer through research. The second reason is that, in the absence of research (that, even though it is not perfect, can at least give us some sense of the truth of a situation, for instance the number of babies affected by a problem) then we tend to look to subjective kinds of knowledge, which include untested theories and our own beliefs.

Some of these theories may turn out to be true, but we cannot know if that is the case. Often they are very intertwined with beliefs, and this is true no matter whether we are talking to someone whose conviction lies with Western medical ideology, one who takes a more holistic view of health or one who holds the view that, as one midwife wrote, *"nature is not haphazard, and is it hard to justify 'correcting' a condition that very likely exists for a reason"* (Kay 2000:19). Other alternative theories include that having relatively low vitamin K levels in utero and early infancy may be beneficial.

We have no idea what the advantage of low vitamin K levels might be, and it's very hard to gather answers to such questions through research, but most of the sensible theories that I have heard tend to be based on the idea that low vitamin K levels may be protective. I do acknowledge that 'sensible' is entirely my own value judgement here. The fact that I think these theories are more sensible than others doesn't automatically make them more likely to be true, but I have also heard some theories that I think are highly unlikely to be true, so that's why I am making a distinction.

Some of these theories simply involve noting that babies' systems are immature and may not be able to handle higher levels of vitamin K at birth, which is why they are born with relatively low levels that they then build up slowly over the first few weeks of their lives, as they become more able to handle higher levels of this substance. Thus, say those who believe this theory, the administration of large amounts of synthetic vitamin K might be problematic.

One researcher published a couple of tantalising studies in the 1990s that looked at possible reasons for low vitamin K levels, variously suggesting that relatively low vitamin K levels may optimise the baby's growth and development both before and after birth (Israels *et al* 1997) and/or be protective against xenobiotics, or foreign substances that may enter the baby's environment and cause potential harm (Israels and Israels 1995).

Other theories relate to the possible advantage of lower vitamin K levels on stem cells. Babies are born with lots of stem cells, which are very special and time-limited cells that can help repair tissues in the days following birth. Some people (including those who market the capture and storage of baby's blood at birth for profit) describe stem cells as being a component of cord blood, but this term is inaccurate. The baby, the cord and the placenta share the same blood. In physics terms, this is a closed system, and the cord can be (among other things) likened to a corridor that transports blood from the baby to the placenta and back again. So 'cord blood' is more accurately termed 'baby's blood' and this is why some people campaign for the cord to be left intact for much longer after birth.

We have now come to realise that, rather than cutting the cord soon after birth, it is better to wait at least 1-3 minutes after the baby is born in order to ensure that a baby gets the additional blood (and thus also stem cells) that they need before their supply is clamped and cut off (WHO 2014). When we wait for at least a minute after a baby is born before clamping the cord, we use the term optimal or delayed cord clamping. The term 'delayed cord clamping' isn't really ideal though, because it can make it sound as if cord clamping is happening later than it would naturally happen. In fact, it is only that we now interfere with the natural process a minute or so later than we previously interfered with it. The act of clamping the cord at any point is an intervention that could be said to interfere with the natural processes that occur within and between the baby and placenta. Some people question the use of the term 'optimal' as well, but that is another discussion.

Once the cord has been clamped and cut, the baby cannot access the blood and stem cells left in the cord. Perhaps babies have lower vitamin K levels than adults because this helps the stem cells to do their job more effectively? I have known parents who believed this to request that vitamin K be given, but given after two weeks rather than at birth. They were concerned that their baby might be at higher-than-average risk so wanted him to receive vitamin K, but they also wanted to give him every chance of experiencing any potential benefits of lower initial vitamin K levels.

A final example of this type of theory is related to our growing knowledge of bacteria and the microbiome. Because our knowledge of this area is in its infancy, I suspect that this is the area that is the most likely to develop and change as we learn more. But the bare bones of this theory at the time of writing relates to our understanding that babies become colonised with bacteria during and after birth. It takes a while for the baby's gut to become colonised with the bacteria it needs for digestion and, among many other things, to synthesise vitamin K from food. This may turn out to be a means of explaining why vitamin K stores take longer to build up, but it doesn't necessarily offer a theory as to why or how this benefits the baby.

Importantly, the medical literature has begun to show evidence of the acknowledgement that low levels of vitamin K may be normal and physiological, at least during pregnancy and at birth. (We will look at the postnatal period shortly). In 2010, for instance, Clarke acknowledged the potential normality of what had previously been deemed to be low levels of vitamin K during the fetal period, stating that, *"very low vitamin K levels in the human fetus appear to be physiological because overt manifestations of antenatal deficiency, such as fetal intracranial haemorrhage, are reported only extremely rarely"*. (2010: 17). Lippi and Francini (2011) have also added to our understanding of this area: *"The haemostatic system is not fully mature until 3 to 6 months of age. It is, therefore, essential to acknowledge that the differences observed between adults and infants are probably physiological and do not always reflect an underlying pathological condition."*

In plain English, these authors are saying that it is probably normal for a baby that the ways in which their body stores and transports blood and blood clotting factors are different from those used by adults.

Although each of the theories discussed here poses a challenge to the idea that babies are deficient in vitamin K, none of the theories are incompatible with Edmund Hey's (2003a) suggestion that, while nature hasn't got it wrong, there is a narrow margin of safety. They do, however, underline why some parents are reluctant to have vitamin K given to their baby, especially in the absence of evidence that their baby is at particular risk. These theories are fuelled by the 'fact' (more on which in a bit) that there are allegedly low levels of vitamin K in breast milk. When people also hear that vitamin K either doesn't cross the placenta well or that the baby doesn't have the substances needed to absorb this (and we are currently not sure whether either of these is true, or whether there is another explanation), this tends to fuel their questioning about whether, for the majority of babies, vitamin K is as necessary in the early weeks of life as they are being told by caregivers. Which in turn begs the question of whether and what harm it might do when given to the population as a whole.

Why do professionals say different things?

As with many areas of health and birth, there exist several different viewpoints, and things can get very confusing. One of these viewpoints is called the technocratic approach. It is also known as the medical model or the obstetric viewpoint in some circles, and I use both of those terms myself sometimes. But as there are a good few doctors who do not subscribe to this viewpoint and plenty of midwives, birth workers, women and families who do, I don't think associating it with a particular professional group is that helpful. Those who hold a technocratic viewpoint tend to place a high value on intervention, technology and drugs. They tend to see women's bodies as fallible and in need of close monitoring and management.

Proponents of the technocratic viewpoint tend to favour hospital birth, birth interventions and universal prophylaxis.

They may be quite risk averse and often favour routine intervention and the idea of saving a few people without necessarily looking at the long-term, psychological, social or other consequences of a treatment or intervention. In other words, they focus on immediate or short-term physical safety, sometimes without considering the bigger picture.

On the other end of the scale is a viewpoint that is more holistic, that sees the body as self-healing and that prioritises a high-touch, low-tech approach. A holistic person or practitioner may see more value in home or out-of-hospital birth and seek to consider alternatives first, although most of those who take a more holistic approach wouldn't rule out Western drugs or treatments when truly warranted. They may be more inclined to favour treating the few people who really do need intervention rather than administering prophylaxis to everybody who might be at risk. Another important element for many proponents of the holistic approach is that decisions are made in relation to the situation and needs of the individual, not the population as a whole. However, it would be remiss of me not to note that there are some dogmatic people within this group as well.

I think it is useful to know that these different approaches exist, and that there are lots of shades of grey in between. It can be confusing to encounter different viewpoints and to feel unsure about who to believe or trust. The key, as in so many things, is that it is often best to read widely (and preferably from published sources and not just blog posts and papers published only on the internet) and to decide for yourself which viewpoint most resonates with your own.

Are there low levels of vitamin K in breast milk?

I have said a lot above about the theory that babies are born with low levels of vitamin K, and I have also discussed specific details of some of the challenges to that theory. The issues are broadly similar when it comes to breast milk. When people first began to question the mass administration of vitamin K, they picked up on the claim of allegedly low levels of vitamin K in breast milk just as much as on the claim of allegedly low levels of vitamin K in babies. But just as babies' vitamin K levels were being compared to adult vitamin K levels – which, as we have seen, may not be an appropriate comparison – we also had no idea of whether the levels of vitamin K in breast milk were accurate, low, too low or just right for the newly born baby. Just as many people baulk at those who challenge the ability of women's bodies to grow and birth their babies, many are also suspicious of those who question the value of breast milk.

The correlation between poor feeding and VKDB was first written about more than 120 years ago:

"The first description of a coagulopathy that had all the attributes of severe vitamin K (VK) deficiency is accredited to a Boston physician, Charles Townsend who in 1894 described 50 cases of a generalized bleeding tendency in neonates, which he thought sufficiently similar to classify as a single entity and which he named the Haemorrhagic Disease of the Newborn (HDN). Townsend noted that HDN could be differentiated from haemophilia by its much earlier time of presentation (usually on days 2 to 3), lack of family history and by its self-limiting time course. Commenting on the complete recovery of one particular 9-day old infant with presumed meningeal haemorrhage, considered by the first physician to be a 'bleeder' (haemophiliac) and a hopeless case, Townsend noted "The belief that the disease was self-limited, with careful artificial and wet nurse feeding, the mother's supply proving a failure, was what saved the baby". Thus Townsend made the first recorded link between the mother's capacity to breastfeed and the haemostatic capacity of her newborn infant." (Shearer 2009)

Lots has changed in our knowledge of breast milk over time, and in the last few years in particular. Those who sought to challenge the low vitamin K allegation when this issue became a hot topic pointed out that it was clearly not appropriate to compare the levels of vitamin K in breast milk with the levels of vitamin K in artificial formula milk. Some people challenged the research upon which this claim was based, pointing out that vitamin K was fat soluble, so would be more likely to be found in colostrum and hindmilk. When put together with the high intervention and relative starvation that was imposed on some babies by the medical profession in the intervening years and the rather rigid feeding regimes at the time when some of this research was carried out, this led to the question of whether there may be more vitamin K in breast milk than was first thought.

As I mentioned earlier, Greer (2004) helped to move our thinking forward in this area when he showed that levels of vitamin K in breast milk were about twice the amount that some of the earlier reports has suggested. He (and others) maintain, however, that vitamin K levels in breast milk are still not high enough for babies. This contrasts with the movement in thinking that has occurred about the so-called low levels of vitamin K that exist in a newborn baby. In a summary of the how the evidence and discussion in this area had evolved over the ten years that had passed since 2003 (when I published the first edition of my booklet for parents on this topic in the UK), I made the observation that, *"When I was reading the literature in the early 2000s, there was an undercurrent of emphasis on the 'low' levels of vitamin K in newborn babies and breast milk. A decade later, I would say that the emphasis has shifted subtly from the 'deficient baby' to the 'dangerous postnatal period', the latter being an alleged source of multiple threats to the breastfed baby's ability to maintain adequate vitamin K stores"*. (Wickham 2013:19).

One important issue is that some of the fundamental ideas around breastfeeding have been challenged, including our ideas about so-called fore and hind milk (Daly *et al* 1993, Hartmann *et al* 1996). We now have a more nuanced knowledge of how breast milk changes over the course of a day and in relation to the needs of an individual baby, which render some of the above arguments moot. Thus, as our knowledge grows and moves on, we need to be open to continually reshaping what we think we know.

I believe that care needs to be taken - by those on all sides of the debate - in the language that is used and the claims that are made in this area. As was discussed in the first part of this book, vitamin K is extremely effective as an intervention. Because artificial milk contains added vitamin K (which means it is a form of oral vitamin K supplementation, albeit not one that is controlled or recommended), it is inevitable that the vast majority of babies who will develop late onset VKDB are those who are exclusively breastfed and whose parents declined a vitamin K supplement at birth. Proponents of mass supplementation argue that these babies are particularly at risk, but this statement isn't helpful, because the statistics illustrate that the vast majority of these babies would be fine even without vitamin K supplementation.

Part of the problem is that we are always looking for clear-cut, black-and-white, all-or-nothing answers. Either breast milk is adequate and good, or it isn't. But the answer might lie in between. Is it so radical to suggest that the amount of vitamin K in the breast milk of a well-nourished woman who is feeding well is adequate for the majority of babies, while acknowledging that there will be exceptions to this? We know from research that the mothers of babies who develop VKDB have normal levels of vitamin K in their milk supply (Shearer 2009). It might be that either these babies aren't getting enough milk, that they have a problem with absorbing the vitamin K from their mother's milk or that some other problem exists which is preventing them from increasing their vitamin K to appropriate levels.

I don't want to move on without pointing out the phrase 'well-nourished' in the previous sentence. This could be important, as we know that many women are not well nourished, for reasons often not of their own making. This is an important issue which professionals should discuss with any woman who is considering not giving vitamin K to her baby. The best dietary source of vitamin K, as on page 32, is dark green leaves such as kale, but maternal supplementation is also an option – see page 30.

In summary, I am arguing that it may be unhelpful to claim that levels of vitamin K in breast milk are too low (which is not true because most babies whose parents decline vitamin K do not develop VKDB) and that it may be just as unhelpful to claim that breast milk is an adequate source of vitamin K for all babies, because this is not true either. Somehow, we need to accept a more nuanced way of looking at this issue which both acknowledges that nature probably does have it right overall but that there exists the occasional baby who will, if vitamin K is not given, experience VKDB.

Why can professional/parent communication be so fraught?

There are a few further things to consider here:

(1) As above, people hold conflicting viewpoints on health care in general and on this topic in particular.

(2) Professionals (and some parents, especially if they have a baby with a particular condition) often become very emotive when it comes to sharing information with others, especially when people consider declining an intervention.

(3) Our culture is very focused on risk and safety, and our health systems tend to prioritise the saving of lives over and above the consequences of interventions. Some professionals worry that, if they do not persuade parents to accept interventions such as vitamin K, they may be sued or otherwise held responsible.

None of this makes the experiences that some parents have had in this area any more acceptable. May and George describe their encounter with a paediatrician:

We had read up on vitamin K and decided not to have it. Ditto some other interventions. Wanted to let the baby have a shot at developing in her own way, but we knew enough to know that we needed to be vigilant and watch the feeding etc. Low tolerance for problems is what our midwife said. No problem with that. We had planned home birth but ended up needing transfer, which was awful enough in itself, but far worse was when we were forced, probably as we had put no vit K on our birth plan, to defend our decision to a senior paediatrician. He came uninvited. Berated us and asked if we wanted our baby to bleed to death. Was it coincidental that he came to see us in the evening when we were tired and our midwife had gone home? He implied that we might not be able to go home the next day if we didn't agree to have the injection. It was awful. We managed to stick to our guns, with thanks to our midwife and some TLC from a lovely care assistant who was on the ward that night, but it was awful.

Sadly, the patriarchal, 'I know best' stance that is often taken in relation to the vitamin K decision can now be seen even in some of the books written by lay people, and it is patronising and counter-productive. To my view, it is better to be honest about the pros and cons, to be clear about what we do and don't know and to be open-minded to different ideas and approaches. I say that not because I want parents to decline vitamin K. I want parents to make the decision that is right for them and their baby, and I want professionals (and those who write on such topics) to treat parents in a respectful manner that acknowledges their intelligence, beliefs and viewpoint and engenders rather than endangers trust. Most parents are entirely capable of making up their own minds about whether or not they want an intervention for their baby and, in fact, many will have decided long before they meet a health care provider.

Heavy-handed persuasion tactics like those described by

May and George and the aggressive language seen in papers such as that by Burke (2013) are not only inappropriate, but they harm relationships and may make it less likely that parents will reach out for help if a problem does occur (Politi *et al* 2017). Although (to my knowledge) we don't have vitamin K-specific research on this topic, a study looking at vaccination decision making showed that parents who declined vaccines reported that their decision was influenced by dissatisfaction with their vaccine discussions with clinicians and the resulting lack of trust in health care professionals (Benin *et al* 2006). Ironically then, those professionals who use heavy-handed tactics to persuade parents that their viewpoint is the correct one may be having the very opposite effect.

Not everyone will agree with what I have just written. Some health services and hospitals set targets for the uptake of things like vitamin K and some birth professionals and educators try to persuade parents to do what they would themselves do. In many cases, they believe that parents should accept vitamin K, but there are also a few who feel it best not to give vitamin K and who seek to persuade parents of this instead.

The authors of some of the papers criticise parents who decide not to give vitamin K, in some cases implying that they are irresponsible. Some state that parental refusal of vitamin K has become more problematic and call upon professionals to work harder at urging parents to accept this for their babies. Professionals who question this or who try to enable informed decision making have experienced bullying and worse.

The effectiveness of vitamin K means that many of the babies who experience VKDB are those whose parents declined vitamin K, and there is often a moral undertone about the fact that an affected baby's parents declined vitamin K at birth, although more often the more confrontational term 'refused' is used (Thomas & Gebara 2004, Brousseau *et al* 2005). Schulte *et al* (2014), for example, responded to the series of cases of VKDB in their hospital by implementing an education programme designed to increase the uptake of vitamin K. Although I have sympathy with their concern that some of the parents of the sick babies had not been made aware of the seriousness of VKDB, there is a substantial difference between seeking to ensure that parents are fully informed but respecting that their decision may be different from ours and trying to bully people into making the decision that someone else thinks is the right one.

3 A pot pourri of FAQs

I have discussed many elements of the vitamin K decision, but a few questions remain. Mostly, unfortunately, they are the ones to which we don't have good answers, but sometimes we can speculate or point to possible further sources of knowledge. The questions and answers in this section have been asked of or sent to me by parents, midwives, doctors or birth workers who have shared the questions that they are most commonly asked or that they themselves would like to know the answer to. Some of these questions have been answered in more detail elsewhere in the book, but they haven't necessarily got a heading of their own, so it is my hope that including shorter answers in this section will make information easier to find.

How is the dosage of vitamin K set?

As is often the case, dosages are set more by what the pharmaceutical companies make and research than because lots of research trials have been carried out to test different preparations and dosages. That said, what we know about dosage and effectiveness of vitamin K is discussed on pages 18 to 23.

Can I ask for my baby to have a smaller dose?

This isn't something that I have known to happen in practice, at least not with injectable vitamin K and babies born at full term. Preterm babies are sometimes given a lower dose, as I discuss on page 66. But that doesn't mean it hasn't happened or couldn't happen with term babies.

With oral vitamin K, the dosage varies widely, so it's common for babies in different areas to receive a variety of dosages at various times. With injectable vitamin K, this would really depend on your care provider, as they would administer the injection, so it would be something to discuss with them.

Standard vitamin K, Konakion MM, is 2mg in 0.2ml, so 1mg in 0.1ml. If a parent wanted a lower dose, it is possible that this could be achieved using 'standard' Konakion MM.

Is it time critical when vitamin K is given?

Yes and no. Vitamin K is not quite as time critical as some drugs or interventions, but it is usually given soon after birth in order to offer maximum protection. But I know of situations where vitamin K has been given a week or two after birth, and it is also given later when given as a treatment for VKDB. There are a few situations when this might happen, for example:

- When parents want to give vitamin K but not immediately (see Olivia's story on page 81).
- When parents initially decline vitamin K but then change their minds.
- When parents initially decline vitamin K but the baby experiences a problem (such as poor feeding) which puts them at higher risk.
- When a baby experiences VKDB and vitamin K is used as a treatment, rather than as a preventative measure.

Why are there follow-up doses with oral vitamin K?

The actual spacing (and volume) of follow-up doses will depend on where you are in the world, but they are spaced in the hope of maximising the effectiveness of the vitamin K. You'll find lots more on this from pages 18 to 23. We know that oral vitamin K isn't quite as effective as injected vitamin K, so we want to do everything we can to maximise its effectiveness. This means spreading the doses out and not giving it on an empty stomach. A number of local factors will affect the timing of this, with one of the main ones being that oral vitamin K is often timed according to when the mother and baby would be seeing a professional for other reasons. This is why there is sometimes a discrepancy between what is ideal and what happens in reality.

Should oral vitamin K always be given with a feed?

Yes. Vitamin K is fat soluble and because of this, as Shearer (2009) points out, *"the absorption of VK is likely to be very poor unless taken with a feed that has bile-salt stimulating properties"*. That includes breast milk or formula.

What is the association between vitamin K and jaundice?

Some midwives and mothers believe that vitamin K can cause or worsen jaundice. Although the midwife who asked me to include this question in the book originally wrote it as *'what is the association between intramuscular vitamin K and jaundice?'*, I have been even more aware over the years of concerns about oral vitamin K and jaundice, so I'll discuss both. What I must say at the outset, however, is that I don't know of any research that has looked into this, so this is purely anecdotal.

I first became aware of this discussion in the early 1990s, when the mass media fuss over vitamin K in the UK caused a number of parents to request that their baby had oral rather than IM vitamin K. In the community midwifery practice where I was working, some of the midwives noticed that they had a number of women and babies who were still receiving home visits at 14 days. They would usually have been discharged from midwifery care ten or eleven days after birth. The midwives looked into this in a relatively informal way (by looking through women's notes while chatting in the community office) and noted that the reason for the delayed discharge in most cases was that the babies were still jaundiced. The midwives began to speculate that, because some of these babies had received oral vitamin K (which had only just become an option and at the time was given at 1, 7 and 28 days), this might be the cause.

I have also heard midwives speculate that the rates of jaundice have increased since IM vitamin K was given. The problem we have with this suggestion, however, is that the midwives (and other professionals) who were around when we first gave vitamin K have pretty much all retired now, and so many other things have changed in women's experiences and midwifery practice that it would be hard to form links even if they were still around to chat with!

The kind of speculation that happens with vitamin K and jaundice is, again, a bit like the concerns that arose in Tennessee, which I discussed from page 16. We can't know if this correlation - and the possible correlations that other midwives and mothers have noted – are indicative of a real change or problem, or whether they are just coincidence. To my knowledge, no-one has looked at these possible links in a systematic way. I always thought it would be interesting to look at the notes of all the women and babies in our community practice and see, for instance, how many babies had oral vitamin K but didn't have jaundice, but that wasn't possible at the time. So we have lots of speculation and stories (which in itself is interesting, because this isn't one isolated hospital) and I know a number of people who make a good case as to why vitamin K may increase the chance of a baby being jaundiced, but we have no research looking at whether there is any link between the two. We also have no reason to think that this jaundice leads to significant or long-term problems.

Is it illegal to decline vitamin K?

No, at least not in the vast majority of countries. I can't speak for those who have very rigid laws and where information isn't easily available to outsiders. It's not illegal to decline vitamin K in the UK, for instance. It's not illegal to decline it in Europe, in Australia or in New Zealand. It's not illegal to decline vitamin K in most US states, but it's a little bit of a grey area in some parts of the USA. Local midwives tell me that, while vitamin K is mandated in some states, such as New York, there is often a way around this.

However, some parents have experienced threats that they will be reported to social services or other government agencies if they decline this or other interventions. There is more information about this on page 85.

How does vitamin K relate to the microbiome?

We're still figuring this out. The word 'microbiome' describes all of the organisms that live on and in our bodies, and by this we mostly mean bacteria that help us to live. I've already discussed a couple of issues related to this. We know that humans make some of their vitamin K in the gut, so the bacteria that live in our digestive systems play a very important part in the production of vital substances such as vitamin K, but we also know that this is a relatively small amount of the total (Shearer 2009, Lippi and Francini 2011) so it may not be that significant; time and research may tell.

Some people are looking to our growing knowledge of the microbiome to help explain why babies are born with relatively low levels of vitamin K, which might help us understand more about normal physiology. Midwives Rachel Reed and Jessie Johnson-Cash (2016) have written a great (and freely available) article on how the microbiome relates to pregnancy, birth and early mothering, but we are still in the early stages of working out whether and how these issues are related. We do know, however, that vitamin K levels may be reduced when people take antibiotics, as Gopakumar *et al* (2010) describe:

"Bacteria in the large intestine produce functional forms of vitamin K. In the absence of dietary vitamin K, small amounts of vitamin K in the large intestine are absorbed passively and prevent severe vitamin K deficiency. This source is eliminated in patients who are on antibiotics, that deplete the intestinal flora capable of vitamin K synthesis. Thus, a common setting of vitamin K deficiency is the case of a patient with inadequate or minimal dietary intake, who is also on treatment with antibiotics."

For this reason, babies who are taking antibiotics or whose mothers take antibiotics during labour may be more at risk from VKDB if they do not receive vitamin K. In some areas of the UK, midwives and birth workers anecdotally report that up to a third of women now receive antibiotics in labour, and midwives working in the US report that the rates are even higher there, so this is a more significant issue than many people think.

Does it make a difference if the baby is born in water?

This is a good question, but as far as I am aware we don't know the answer. Some people wonder if being born in water changes the baby's microbiome so that it makes more or less vitamin K, but we really do not know.

Does the type of birth affect VKDB risk?

At one time, it was thought that babies who had a traumatic birth (which some people would say was more likely with an instrumental birth) were at higher risk of a bleed. But no evidence has been found to support this theory. We also know that babies born at home or in birth centres are among those who get VKDB so we no longer think there is a link.

Does optimal cord clamping affect vitamin K?

This is another great question to which I can only offer the frustrating answer that we don't know. We do know that it is better for the baby to receive their full complement of blood for other reasons (as discussed on page 47).

One of the main theories about why babies might need low levels of vitamin K relates to the benefits of stem cells, and babies get more stem cells with optimal (or delayed) cord clamping. But we don't know whether this will lead to the baby having more vitamin K. Furthermore, the stem cell theory attempts to explain why the relatively low level of vitamin K might be beneficial so this is something that we need to think about carefully and carry out research into. But again, optimal cord clamping does provide many other benefits and is well worth doing for other reasons.

What about vitamin K and preterm babies?

Babies who are born earlier than average are seen as a higher risk group, and it is thought that preterm babies have less vitamin K than term babies (Pilcher and Pilcher 2008). In fact, there has been little research into this, as discussed by Ardell *et al* (2010):

"VKDB in preterm infants has not been extensively discussed in the literature. In part, this may be because most preterm infants admitted to neonatal intensive care units are given prophylactic Vitamin K (often without parental input) and because parenteral nutrition is started early in the hospital course and provides preterm infants with more than enough vitamin K. However, there are a variety of reasons to believe that preterm infants may be at greater risk of vitamin K deficiency bleeding and that this bleeding may be of greater consequence, particularly regarding the risk of intraventricular haemorrhage." (Ardell *et al* 2010).

One of the increased risks comes from the fact that many preterm babies are given antibiotics, which increase the chance of VKDB. However, Costakos *et al* (2003) highlighted concerns about preterm babies receiving higher levels of vitamin K than was ideal and, in 2010, Greer (one of Costakos' co-authors on the original paper) again reiterated how, because of multiple sources of vitamin K intake, preterm babies can end up with vitamin serum concentrations a hundred times higher than those found in adults and ten to twenty times greater than those found in term formula-fed infants (who are already receiving considerable daily supplementation). Both papers argued that this warrants further study and/or changes to the nutrition that preterm babies receive. Some units have different protocols for preterm babies, but by no means all, and it is worrying that an issue first raised in the literature in 2003 still does not seem to have received widespread attention.

What is the impact of oral vitamin K on the newborn gut considering the recommendations for exclusive breastfeeding?

Great question. We have no idea what the answer is, though, but many people are concerned about how oral vitamin K may impact the gut and microbial development of the newborn. We are really only just beginning to learn about the microbiome and how it alters during and after birth, feeding and the early days and weeks of a baby's life (Reed and Johnson-Cash 2016). One thing we do know is that having a vaginal birth and being breastfed gives babies the best chance of developing their good bacteria and it would appear that babies who have these advantages are able to better protect themselves against disease. Substances other than breast milk can disturb the growth of good bacteria, and this is why some people are concerned about whether oral vitamin K may interfere with microbial development, especially in babies who are otherwise only having breast milk. But, as with so many other questions relating to this topic, we don't have enough knowledge to know for sure. This is one of the areas in which our knowledge is likely to grow significantly over the next few years.

How useful is it for women to significantly increase their intake of vitamin K in pregnancy?

I've written about this on pages 30-32, so please check there for more detailed information. The bottom line is that vitamin K doesn't cross the placenta very well, so while it's always good to eat well and include lots of dark leaves in one's diet, eating lots of vitamin K-rich foods while pregnant doesn't seem to make much difference to the baby's level of vitamin K. There seems to be more value in taking vitamin K supplements (or possibly increasing dietary vitamin K, though I have not seen research on this) while breastfeeding, but no research has been carried out to look at whether this is effective as a means of preventing VKDB.

Would eating the placenta increase vitamin K levels?

Another very interesting question! Unfortunately, we don't know for sure whether or how eating the placenta might affect vitamin K levels. If I had come across any specific research – or even discussion – on this topic in the midwifery or medical literature, then I would have added it into this book, but I have never seen anything written on this. There are a few things we do know that are related however, and they all seem to point to the conclusion that eating the placenta probably wouldn't have much effect.

We know, for instance, that meat contains vitamin K, although it is not such a good source of vitamin K as green leafy vegetables. We don't think that vitamin K can cross the placenta easily, and this is thought to be one possible reason for babies having relatively low levels of vitamin K, though it is also possible that vitamin K does cross the placenta but the baby doesn't have the substances needed to absorb it. So there may not be much vitamin K in the placenta to begin with. We should remember that the placenta is the baby's tissue rather than the mother's tissue, so the levels of vitamin K in the placenta are likely to be similar to the levels in the baby, which we know are comparatively low.

Finally, if we assume (and it is a total assumption, because I cannot find data on this) that the placenta contains the same amount of vitamin K as, say, liver (which is the meat that those who have eaten their placenta say it is most like) then one average placenta would contain about 1mg of vitamin K. As I discussed on page 30, we know that women need to ingest 5mg of vitamin K per day in order to confer what researchers consider an adequate level of protection to their baby through their breast milk. Therefore, as women only have one placenta, eating it is unlikely to make a difference in respect of the baby's vitamin K levels.

Is there a way to screen a baby's blood at one week of age or later to confirm that clotting factors have risen adequately?

Not that I know of, but you may wish to ask your midwife or doctor as this may vary around the world. Private vitamin K tests are available in some areas, but they are expensive and laboratories may be reluctant to take blood from small babies. There are other tests to investigate unexplained bleeding or bruising or to monitor the ability of someone's blood to coagulate, or clot, but these are not generally available outside of a hospital or other clinical setting.

One key issue is that we do not have good knowledge about what the normal levels of vitamin K are at different stages for babies who do not receive vitamin K. We haven't carried out a study measuring babies' vitamin K levels over time and we have treated the vast majority of babies with vitamin K for many years. So it would be hard to interpret the results of any testing. Another concern would be the fact that, like with many screening tests, a normal or healthy result on one occasion couldn't be taken as a guarantee that the baby would maintain adequate vitamin K levels after that, for instance if breastfeeding difficulties developed.

If we decline vitamin K at birth, can we have it later?

Yes, and most professionals would be happy to arrange this for you. VKDB occurs only in the first few months of a baby's life, so if your baby is more than about 4 months old you may find you are told that it would no longer be beneficial, as your baby is likely to be able to maintain their own vitamin K stores by that point.

How do we know if a baby has been protected?

There is no way of knowing this. Although vitamin K is very effective, nothing is one hundred percent effective and there is no test available to determine whether a baby is or is not protected or at lower/higher risk than average.

Does vitamin K contain animal products?

In some versions, yes, but not in every form. Some forms of vitamin K contain an excipient called glycocholic acid, and some pharmaceutical companies make this from the gall bladders of cattle. Lecithin may also be derived from animals or eggs, though it can also be made from plants. But pharmaceutical companies may change the formulation of preparations or the source of the ingredients, so the only way of knowing for sure is to check the product information sheet and/or contact the manufacturer.

What is the relationship between vitamin K and liver disease?

Late onset VKDB is often associated with undiagnosed cholestasis (or liver disease) which prevents vitamin K from being properly absorbed. The baby can then experience bleeding as a result of the poor absorption. When a baby with undiagnosed liver disease is given prophylactic vitamin K at birth, however, this can also, as Emma's story illustrates on page 75, mask the diagnosis of the liver disease, which can have negative consequences for the treatment of the affected baby.

4 Parents' experiences

Like the first booklet that I wrote on this topic, this book has been written in the hope of helping parents to become more informed and able to make the decisions that are right for them, so it is only right that we should return to this question at the end. The vitamin K decision continues to be a difficult one for some parents, principally because our lack of knowledge about which babies might benefit from vitamin K leaves a fairly stark choice. Sadly, some fairly unhelpful attitudes persist, especially when parents make the choice to decline vitamin K. Clarke and Shearer's (2007) suggestion to professionals epitomises what happens to many parents in practice, at least in the UK:

"We believe refusal should trigger involvement of a senior paediatrician to explore parental concerns and discuss all available options. Infants who suffered VKDB not uncommonly feature among medicolegal cases so meticulous documentation is imperative." (Clarke & Shearer 2007: 743)

Sometimes, such discussions are friendly and simply ensure that the parents have all the relevant information. More often, they are confrontational, accusatory and/or designed to persuade parents that their decision is irresponsible and they should comply with the paediatrician's recommended course of action, which is almost always to give vitamin K. A childbirth educator heard a paediatrician saying to parents, *"If you loved your baby as much as I love babies, you would give your baby vitamin K."* The use of such statements is a form of emotional blackmail which occurs far too often, and the suggestion that parents might not love their baby as much as a health professional is both shocking and deeply offensive.

Not long after the very first version of this book was published, two articles appeared in the British publications *Midwifery Matters* (Neiger 2004) and *AIMS Journal* (Bevan

2003). Both of these articles discussed how women often received little information on this topic and frequently did not realise that they even had a choice about whether or not their baby received vitamin K. While this situation has changed in many areas, it still always strikes me when I look for updates in the literature on this topic that there is so little research exploring what parents want or need. There is also almost nothing in the professional literature that shares parents' views or voices. I found one study that set out to evaluate the acceptability of a new regimen of oral vitamin K and concluded that this regimen is well tolerated and acceptable to parents (Strehle *et al* 2010). Yet the researchers had not asked parents for their views. Instead, they had only sought midwives' perceptions of parents' views. I found this odd because, while many midwives will be very keen to understand and respond to parents' concerns, it is hard to see how researchers can justify the claim that parents find something acceptable when the parents haven't actually been asked for their views. This isn't unique, though.

Because I do feel it is vital to ask for and include parents' stories and voices, this section begins with a handful of stories that have been shared with me by parents and midwives. (For the record, I didn't deliberately exclude fathers or co-parents; I just didn't receive any responses from them, other than the story shared by May and George on page 55 and Paul's question (page 38). I'd be happy to include additional responses in future books, and anyone interested in sharing their story can reach me via my website, www.sarawickham.com).

In some ways, several of these are unusual stories and their inclusion doesn't reflect the fact that the decisions these parents are making are common. But I have tried to ensure that I share stories from different perspectives, and that each one has something useful to teach or to enable readers to think about.

Emma's story

I have two children. The eldest was born via caesarean section after a long, non-progressing induction for being post-dates, and after reading the handouts and attending antenatal classes, we consented to giving her oral vitamin K. My second was a lovely term VBAC, with a shoulder dystocia (easily resolved), and we opted to give oral vitamin K again as that was what we did the first time around.

When the youngest was 13 days old I noticed a little bruise in the middle of a chub roll on her thigh. I figured we must have bumped it or something, then the next day we saw/felt that she had a big bump on her clavicle, so decided to see our GP. The day before we were able to see the GP I found another wee bruise at the bottom of her ribs, and the following morning another bruise on her back.

The GP thought the clavicle was from it being broken (from getting stuck on the way out), and she thought the bruises were odd as they each had a wee bump in the middle, so she referred us to the hospital to get checked out.

So we went in, and they did some blood tests. Her INR (clotting) came back as 9 (off the charts high), the doctors said it was because we had given her the oral vitamin k rather than the intramuscular dose (she'd had the 2 scheduled oral doses, with the third and final due in 2 weeks). The doctors asked why we had only given her the oral and didn't we know it didn't do anything.

Then her liver function tests came back abnormal and they started looking at liver disease. At one point they were thinking she had biliary atresia [a disease in which the bile ducts are blocked], and the doctor admitted it was good that she hadn't had the intramuscular vitamin K as then her clotting would have been ok and we wouldn't have picked up that she was unwell. For biliary atresia there is a surgery that they can do that greatly delayed the need of a liver transplant if done before 6 weeks old...

After spending 4 weeks on the children's ward, having numerous blood tests, a HIDA scan and an x-ray, they ruled out a lot of things, but still had no diagnosis. They did a liver biopsy and found out she had Progressive Familial Intrahepatic Cholestasis, in the end she had a liver transplant at 11 months old, and has been doing extremely well since!

I do not regret not giving my daughter(s) intramuscular vitamin K, in fact if I had any more children I would chose not to give them any vitamin K - my daughter who had liver disease and blood that actually wasn't clotting (despite 2 doses of oral vitamin k (which the liver disease would have hindered her absorbing)) did not bleed out, nor did she bleed where there was trauma to her clavicle despite breaking it at birth. Maybe she was lucky? Maybe not? Maybe our babies are not flawed? Maybe our babies do not need very high levels of vitamin K for their blood to clot effectively?

Late onset VKDB, occurring between the ages of 2 and 12 weeks has a 1 in 15,000 to 1 in 20,000 chance, and this is where the babies with liver disease or malabsorption issues are at particular risk. If we are giving all babies intramuscular vitamin K, how many of those babies have other issues going on (like liver disease) that could have been identified earlier, which affects their outcomes (as in biliary atresia, where the earlier the diagnosis then the higher the chance that liver transplant can be delayed)?

Are we too readily giving babies vitamin K?

I feel it is important to know that even if you do all the tests, if you do everything prophylactically, that you can still have an unexpected outcome. If you choose to give your baby vitamin K your baby may still have bleeding issues and it is important to know the signs to look out for whether or not you chose to give it. Know that if you decline, that you can change your mind at any time. Know that we don't know the long-term effects of giving our babies synthetic vitamin K. Follow your instincts, and keep going until they are satisfied.

Anna's story

Yes, it's rare, but unfortunately there isn't a way of telling in advance which babies might be affected by VKDB, and that was the most important thing for us. The leukaemia link was never proven and now different things are used in the shot. I think the injection is the way to go and all of mine had it. They are healthy 24, 23, 19 and 16-year-olds. No ill consequences that I can see. I would give it again.

Cybele's story

We decided not to give Emily vitamin K when we learned how rare VKDB was. I was the same with testing for group B strep (GBS) bacteria; just not interested when I saw the statistics. In both cases, we're talking about something really rare and yes, I know it can be fatal and yes I know she could have been the one in twelve thousand, or even more rare with GBS, I think, but what would the consequences of giving vitamin K or taking antibiotics be?

People say you'll do anything to protect your baby, and of course you will, but it's no good only thinking one dimensionally.

We could be trading a possible risk of something rare and serious for a more likely risk of interfering with her physiology or growth. How would that protect her? Both must have effects on their tiny bodies, and if nature meant for babies to have that much vitamin K then I'm thinking that they would either be born with it or we would have gallons in our breast milk.

I was lucky. I had a home birth with an independent [midwife], but I came under pressure later from the health visitor. What helped me cope with pressure from her was to just kind of allow her to rant on and just keep saying, "thank you, I just want a day or two more to think about it" rather than saying an outright no which felt like it would trigger a response that would put more pressure on me. Then I waited til Dave was there before we gave the final decision. The feminist in me is a bit embarrassed at that, but I felt I needed the moral support because I was worried that she would go on more. That was the one bit that marred the experience, actually. Being made to feel as if we were irresponsible when, actually, we had thought really long and hard about it, probably more than most people.

Ella's story

Jack was born in the hospital and I didn't want to take any chances so yes, we had the vitamin K. I don't see why you wouldn't, as they can die if you don't. We did most things they suggested. They are the experts, so they know best. I was happy with the care we received.

Aisha's story

It was given orally to both of my girls. After I gave birth to the first they didn't mention an injection, not so far as I can remember. I'm sure I would remember. The second one they didn't even ask me. I wasn't in the room and they asked my husband and I was not OK with that, but what can you do? I would have had the injection if they had asked me. It was so much hassle getting the oral drops every few weeks, I had to go to the doctors', but the injection they just give once and then it's done.

Jo's story

For one of my babies born at home, I opted for vitamin K drops as I was convinced that the standard injection would be an unnecessarily traumatic intervention for my newborn baby, with little obvious benefit. I made this decision before the birth and communicated this clearly. Once I'd given birth, however, that decision was overlooked as I was offered the standard vitamin K injection for my baby. I refused this offer, and explained that I wanted to have the oral drops instead. It would have been much easier for me at that stage, however, to have simply accepted the injection being offered.

Over the course of subsequent home visits, my request for oral drops was repeatedly the cause of confusion, as each new midwife who visited had to be told again about this request. Eventually a prescription was ordered for the drops, and my husband was able to collect them (walking a couple of miles in the pouring rain to do so, as we live in a village without a chemist and at that time had no car). For me, this was an interesting - if minor - example of how the system resists requests outside of the standard model. So if women want drops, I'd strongly suggest that they should be warned that they may need to make some effort to get them.

A further irony is that I have now decided that even the drops represent an unnecessary intervention, and one that is potentially MORE harmful than the injection, in terms of how it interferes with the benefits to the baby achieved from exclusive breastfeeding. I thought that I was a fairly savvy consumer of maternity services by the time I was onto baby number 4, but I now realise that it's just so easy to get drawn into choosing from the limited menu of options offered by the NHS on any given issue, rather than considering more broadly whether or not any of the options offered are actually what you want for yourself and your baby. My choice now would be to opt out of the vitamin K programme altogether.

Martha's story

I declined the vitamin K injection for both of my babies and with the first gave her vitamin K orally.

With my second I had taken a look at the evidence again and decided that we wouldn't give it at all after birth. However, at three weeks she was admitted to hospital with a fever and had to be given intravenous antibiotics for a week.

Being a little paranoid I looked into whether there was any problem that she hadn't had vitamin K and decided this wasn't any issue. Unfortunately, at one stage there was an issue with the doctor inserting a cannula and to calm my baby down they suggested I squeeze glucose into her mouth via a little plastic tube. This must have nicked her mouth slightly (although I hadn't felt it had) as suddenly I realised there was some blood in her mouth. I pointed this out to doctor and he immediately asked me if she'd had vitamin K at birth. I had to admit she hadn't.

For me it brought into sharp relief the decisions we make and in a week of having an ill baby I suddenly really regretted not giving her the vitamin K injection (I felt if she'd just had it at birth it would be one thing less I needed to worry about). The doctor asked me if she hadn't been offered it or if I had decided not for her to be given it. I said it was the latter and in that moment realised that I wouldn't really have had a strong conviction for her not to have had it other than my instinct.

None of us felt that the bleeding in her mouth was vitamin K related, however as a precaution a consultant recommend that I give her the oral doses. I did this but wasn't quite sure why and wasn't even sure what impact it would have at that stage. I was feeling guilty and would have done anything to be sure my baby would be OK.

Olivia's story

As a midwife, I once cared for a lady who made a choice I had never thought about with regard to vitamin K prophylaxis for her baby. She had a child already, who had inadvertently been given a massive overdose of vitamin K (not in the UK), and experienced a stroke in the neonatal period which had left her with weakness on one side. No one was willing to say it was or wasn't because of the vitamin K. She had a PhD, so was very confident in analysing research papers and making decisions. Her choice was to have the vitamin K prophylaxis given to the baby intramuscularly at discharge from midwifery care, which because she had independent midwifery care was when the baby was a few weeks old (not at 10 days like in the NHS). Her rationale was that early onset VKDB was almost always associated with maternal conditions or medications; medium onset was usually mild, but late onset was the one to be slightly worried about. She went on to have another baby, this time within NHS maternity care, and made the same decision again.

5 Signposting the roads less travelled

One big concern I have about our current approach to health care is the way that we tend to offer or recommend just one pathway, with the result that any parents who decide to step off it or consider other options are pretty much then on their own. That might mean that they spend hours searching the internet without any guidance as to the variable quality of information out there, only to be later criticised for accessing poor-quality debate. It can mean that they have trouble exercising their right to decide what's right for their baby.

But possibly worse than that, it can mean that they may be caring for a baby who has a tiny chance of developing VKDB but without having any useful information about when to seek help, what might alter that risk and the other things that might be useful for them to know. These issues are addressed in this section of the book. The only reason there is not a long section in this book called 'How to get vitamin K if you decide to have it' is because there is absolutely no need for it at all – that's an easy path to navigate, and so I am saving trees (or, OK, e-reader batteries) by making that a very short section.

If you decide to have vitamin K for your baby

Talk to your care provider. They will almost certainly be very happy to help make this happen. In the unlikely event that they do not feel this way, look for another care provider.

If you decide you want vitamin K for your baby, but in a modified or unusual way, or perhaps at a different time

Still talk to your care provider, but it's probably best to do some research first. Depending on who your care provider is, and what your relationship with them is like, you may need to be prepared to explain or defend your request. Your care provider might feel challenged by your ideas, or they might share some or all of your views or concerns but feel unable to challenge the system. They might be really supportive. If you find you do not agree on the first conversation, thank them for their time and let them know that you would like some time to consider your decision. You may wish to ask them whether they could refer you to someone else who might feel able to support your decision. There is lots of further advice in the next section that might also help.

If you decide to decline vitamin K, or to 'wait and see'

Again, talk to your care provider. It can be helpful (if it is true) to point out that, like many of the parents who decline vitamin K, you are not saying that you will never let vitamin K pass your baby's skin or lips. Many parents who do not want routine prophylaxis will reconsider this decision if there is particular cause for concern or if their baby appears to have VKDB, and this can be a useful conversation to have with your care provider. In other words, it can be useful to let anyone who questions your decision or considers it to be unreasonable know if you are saying 'not now' rather than 'not ever'. Be aware that some people may (correctly) tell you that VKDB is not always predictable.

As I have now mentioned several times, some parents find themselves being pressured or coerced by professionals, and in some areas of the world parents may even be threatened or sanctioned for declining interventions such as vitamin K. In the UK, parents are concerned that their child may be put on the 'at risk' register, and many other countries have similar sanctions involving social services or the police. This kind of situation can be extremely unpleasant, but such situations are really uncommon. Many parents ask where they can get help if they decline vitamin K and find that their midwife or doctor or the baby's paediatrician is insisting it is essential.

It can be really valuable to seek support from other parents, friends and family. Sometimes, the pressure to make decisions and your ability to resist consenting to something that you do not want is made harder by the fact that you are tired and overwhelmed with being a new parent and recovering from pregnancy and birth. This applies to all parents.

If you have supportive people around you, it can be helpful to ask friends or family members to be with you in a situation where you are concerned that you may be pressured or asked to make a decision that you do not want to make. If you do not have family nearby, or your family is not supportive, there may be parents' groups, websites or organisations who can offer support.

Professionals and birth workers can also be a good source of support although, if you are reading this book in order, you will now know that professionals do not all agree on this issue! Some clinicians (and some lay commentators) are very certain that all babies should have vitamin K and feel it is OK to try and coerce people, and some are certain that it is not a good thing. These folk may also be coercive, but in a different way. Many people, though, are open to having a conversation about the pros and cons and are honest about what we do and don't know while being more supportive of parents' right to make this decision for themselves. Seek out the latter kind, ideally early in pregnancy. This means that you are more likely to get the kind of care that you want and deserve throughout pregnancy, birth and afterwards. If you do not feel comfortable with your care provider at any stage, then do everything you can to change to someone else. In the UK, it is your right to change your caregiver.

As one of the women who shared their story for this book said, it is important to trust your instincts. Even if you are in a country where you do not get a choice or if you only realised after giving birth that you have a provider who does not share or support your views, you may still have the option of asking for another caregiver. It is worth asking friends and fellow parents who they would recommend. And if you encounter someone wonderful, then tell all your friends about them!

As well as midwives, you may also find supportive doctors and doulas. Independent childbirth educators can be a good source of information, as they often learn about who is most willing and able to help and support parents in different situations.

Finally, although I can't list the situation in every country from which people will read this book, there are a growing number of organisations, resources and people who will help you to gather local knowledge. There is a fabulous book in the UK called *Am I Allowed?*, which has been written by Beverley Beech (2014) and which I would thoroughly recommend for anyone making birth-related decisions. The charities *Birthrights* (www.birthrights.org.uk) and *AIMS* (www.aims.org.uk) have useful websites with good information about women's and parents' legal rights in relation to maternity care in the UK. There are similar organisations in other countries, and the internet is a good way to find them. As before, independent childbirth educators can be a good source of information and support.

Although I am unable to answer individual queries on this or other topics, I do have a website (which you can find at www.sarawickham.com), a free newsletter and social media pages on which I post new research and thinking and which you are welcome to use or subscribe to in order to get up-to-date information and connect with others. If you're a midwife, birth worker or educator interested in helping others to understand more about this topic, I also run online courses on this topic that you might enjoy and find useful – more on that on my website too.

Changing your mind

If you are considering declining vitamin K, it can be useful to think through whether there are circumstances in which you would change your mind. Some of the situations in which parents might reconsider their decision to give vitamin K at birth include their baby being born prematurely, being unwell or experiencing problems (such as birth asphyxia) during birth. Other examples include situations in which a baby's mother is taking certain kinds of medication or if there are immediate feeding problems. These are all good reasons to reconsider whether vitamin K might be useful at or around the time of birth.

Things to watch for

Assuming that vitamin K is not given at birth (or within a short time of birth), there are a few more things that we know about which babies are most likely to end up with VKDB and why. I believe it is helpful to share this information with parents who are considering declining (or who have declined) vitamin K. This ensures that they know when and why to seek help.

We have already seen some useful summaries that offer helpful information. The key issues that we are looking for include:

- Feeding difficulties (because babies who have feeding problems, even when they are a few months old, may not be able to maintain their vitamin K stores).
- Signs of liver disease (because of the babies who develop VKDB, many do so in conjunction with liver disease).
- Signs of bruising or bleeding (because these are signs of VKDB).

We can translate this knowledge into a few concrete tips and suggestions. These will not help identify every baby who is at risk of a serious bleed, as it is estimated that about a third of babies show no prior symptoms, but it may help reduce the incidence and severity of problems in some babies. If you are worried about a baby, seek help immediately, as the earlier a problem is detected, the more likely it is that treatment will be effective.

- **Respond quickly to feeding problems.**
  - Parents and caregivers should have a low threshold for responding to any feeding issues in a baby who has not had vitamin K.
  - If babies do not feed well at birth and in the first day or two of life, they will quickly exhaust their vitamin K reserves. Parents who have declined vitamin K may wish to reconsider giving IM or oral vitamin K if their baby does not establish feeding within this time frame.
  - This applies on an ongoing basis as well as in the hours after birth. Babies are deemed to be at risk of VKDB until at least 3-4 months of age. Some of the babies who develop VKDB are those who have not established breastfeeding quite as well as others. They may have managed to get enough milk for their nutritional needs, but not enough to build and store appropriate levels of vitamin K.

- **Look out for bleeding or bruising.**
  - In a baby who has not received vitamin K, any bruising or bleeding should be investigated. Bruising may appear anywhere on the body and can be hidden in skin folds or creases. Bleeding may occur from the umbilical cord site, nose or mouth, or you may see blood in the baby's nappy (diaper). The baby's poo may be dark or black in appearance, although this should not be confused with meconium, the tar-like substance that fills the baby's bowels during pregnancy and is expelled during the first couple of days of life.

- **Be aware of the other signs of VKDB.**
  - Babies who have VKDB may also vomit (throw up), be fussier or more sleepy than usual, have seizures (fits) or have visible bulging around a fontanelle (the soft spot on their head). Any such symptoms require <u>immediate</u> medical help. It is also important to assess babies who 'fail to thrive' or have diarrhoea.

- **Be aware that antibiotics deplete vitamin K stores**
  - Antibiotics interfere with the body's back-up supply of vitamin K (Gopakumar 2010). Re-evaluate the need for external vitamin K if antibiotics are taken by mother or baby. This includes antibiotics given in labour and, as with all these points, it continues to apply for the first few months of the baby's life.

- **Seek help for jaundice**
  - Many babies have jaundice in the few days after birth. But later or persistent jaundice can also indicate a liver problem, which increases the risk of VKDB. All parents should be on the lookout for jaundice, even if vitamin K has been given.
  - Be vigilant for other symptoms of liver problems, such as dark urine or light-coloured faeces.

- **If a baby needs medical care of any kind, let care providers know that vitamin K was not given.**
  - Some parents are understandably reluctant to do this, because they fear that they may face rebuke or persuasion to give vitamin K. But if a baby is experiencing a problem related to low vitamin K, then it is important that caregivers know this, not least because giving vitamin K can quickly reverse some problems before they worsen.

A final word

I often get funny looks when I spend ages telling parents everything I know about a topic and then follow that up by asking them not to take my word for it. But I still do it, regardless, and there are a few reasons for that.

One is that I want every parent to make the decision that is right for them, and not what they think I or the local paediatrician or the family next door would do. So a good way to figure out what you think and need and want is to cast your net about for a few different opinions. Nobody can be truly objective, and even those of us who consciously try to give a balanced viewpoint will put more emphasis on some things and less on others. If you seek a few opinions, you'll hopefully get a good overall picture. Though yes, you can also get confused, so you'll need to use your judgment.

The second reason is that I don't want you to believe everything you read, and that goes especially for what you read on the internet. But it would be unhelpfully inconsistent, I think, to say, *'hey, treat everything else with caution, but what I'm saying is fine'*. And I don't want to be inconsistent, so please go ahead and treat my views and analysis with scepticism as well. Just please be sure to apply the same scepticism when you read what journalists and others write about this area!

Finally, things change. I am really aware, for instance, that much of what I wrote when I first became interested in this topic is now out of date. Some of what is written in the older work on this area is now inaccurate. I have discussed this with colleagues who were undertaking research at the same time, and we marvel at how our understanding of this area has grown. What we wrote wasn't inaccurate at the time, but I met Laura and began my own vitamin K journey more than twenty years ago now, and knowledge and understanding move on. That's not a bad thing; it means our knowledge is growing. And it will continue to grow, so do be open to other, newer ideas if you spot them. Because at the end of the day, what matters most is that you make the decision that's right for you and your baby and your family. It's your path to find, and I wish you well in finding it.

References

Ansell P, Bull D, Roman E (1996). Childhood leukaemia and intramuscular vitamin K: findings from a case-control study. British Medical Journal, 313: 204-05.

Ansell P, Roman E, Fear NT *et al* (2004). Vitamin K update: survey of paediatricians in the UK. British Journal Midwifery 12(1): 38-41.

Ardell S, Offringa M and Soll R (2010). Prophylactic vitamin K for the prevention of vitamin K deficiency bleeding in preterm neonates. Cochrane protocol. DOI: 10.1002/14651858.CD008342

Beech BAL (2014). Am I Allowed? London: AIMS.

Benin AL, Wisler-Scher DJ, Colson E *et al* (2006). Qualitative analysis of mothers' decision making about vaccines for infants: the importance of trust. Pediatrics. 117(5):1532-41.

Bevan V (2003). Vitamin K in Lincoln: consumer choice or no voice? AIMS Journal 15(3): 18-20.

Bolisetty S, Gupta JM, Graham GG (1998). Vitamin K in preterm breastmilk with maternal supplementation. Acta Paediatrica 87(9): 960-62.

Brousseau TJ, Kissoon N, McIntosh B (2005). Vitamin K deficiency mimicking child abuse. Journal Emergency Medicine 29(3): 283-88.

Burke C (2013). Vitamin K deficiency bleeding: overview and considerations. Journal of Pediatric Health Care.

Busfield A, McNinch A, Tripp J (2007). Neonatal vitamin K prophylaxis in Great Britain and Ireland: the impact of perceived risk and product licensing on effectiveness. Archives of Disease in Childhood 92(9): 754-58.

Busfield A, Samuel R, McNinch A *et al* (2012). Vitamin K Deficiency Bleeding After NICE Guidance and Withdrawal of Konakion

Neonatal: British Paediatric Surveillance Unit Study, 2006-2008. Archives of Disease in Childhood 98 (1), 41-47.

Cancer Research UK (2017). Leukaemia (all subtypes combined) incidence statistics. http://www.cancerresearchuk.org/health-professional/cancer-statistics/statistics-by-cancer-type/leukaemia/incidence

Centers for Disease Control and Prevention (CDC) (2013). Notes from the field: late vitamin K deficiency bleeding in infants whose parents declined vitamin K prophylaxis — Tennessee, 2013. Morbidity and Mortality Weekly Report 62(45): 901.

Clarke P, Shearer MJ (2007). Vitamin K deficiency bleeding: the readiness is all. Archives of Disease in Childhood 92(9): 741-43.

Clarke P (2010). Vitamin K prophylaxis for preterm infants. Early Human Development 86(1 suppl): 17-20.

Costakos DT, Greer FR, Love LA et al (2003). Vitamin K prophylaxis for premature infants: 1 mg versus 0.5 mg. American Journal of Perinatology. 20: 485–90.

Cranford M (2011). Vitamin K: did nature get it right? Midwifery Today 98: 28,66.

Daly SEJ, DiRosso A, Owens RA et al (1993). Degree of breast emptying explains changes in the fat content, but not fatty acid composition, of human milk. Experimental Physiology 78:741-55.

Danielsson N, Hoa DP, Thang NV et al (2004). Intracranial haemorrhage due to late onset vitamin K deficiency bleeding in Hanoi province, Vietnam. Archives of Disease in Childhood: Fetal and Neonatal Edition 89(6): F546-50.

Darlow B and Harding J (1995). Vitamin K prophylaxis in the newborn. New Zealand Medical Journal 108: 514.

Darlow BA, Phillips AA, Dickson NP (2011). New Zealand surveillance of neonatal vitamin K deficiency bleeding (VKDB): 1998-2008. Journal of Paediatrics and Child Health 47(7): 460-64.

Dekker R (2014). Evidence on: The Vitamin K Shot in Newborns. https://evidencebasedbirth.com/evidence-for-the-vitamin-k-shot-in-newborns/

Enkin M, Kierse, MJNC, Neilson J *et al* (2002). Effective Care in Pregnancy and Childbirth. 3rd Edition. Oxford University Press.

Golding J, Greenwood R, Birmingham K *et al* (1992). Childhood cancer, intramuscular vitamin K, and pethidine given during labour. British Medical Journal 305(6849): 341–346.

Gopakumar H, Sivji R, and Rajiv PK (2010). Vitamin K deficiency bleeding presenting as impending brain herniation Journal of Pediatric Neuroscience 5(1): 55–58.

Greer FR, Marshall SP, Foley AL *et al* (1997). Improving the vitamin K status of breastfeeding infants with maternal vitamin K supplements. Pediatrics 99(1):88-92.

Greer FR (2004). Vitamin K in human milk — still not enough. Acta Paediatrica 93(4): 449-50.

Greer FR (2010). Vitamin K the basics — what's new? Early Human Development 86(1 suppl): 43-7.

Guala A, Guarino R, Zaffaroni M *et al* (2005). The impact of national and international guidelines on newborn care in the nurseries of Piedmont and Aosta Valley, Italy. BMC Pediatrics 5(45).

Hansen KN, Minousis M, Ebbesen F (2003). Weekly oral vitamin K prophylaxis in Denmark. Acta Paediatrica 92(7): 802-05.

Hartmann PE, Owens RA, Cox DB *et al* (1996) Breast development and control of milk synthesis. Food and Nutrition Bulletin 17(4): 292-302.

Harvey B (2008). Newborn vitamin K prophylaxis: developments and dilemmas. British Journal of Midwifery 16(8): 516-19.

Hey E (2003a). Vitamin K — can we improve on nature? MIDIRS Midwifery Digest 13(1): 7-12.

Hey E (2003b). Vitamin K — what, why, and when. Archives of Disease in Childhood: Fetal and Neonatal Edition 88(2): F80-83.

Heubi JE, Setchell KDR, Jha P *et al* (2014). Treatment of bile acid amidation defects with glycocholic acid. Hepatology. 61(1): 268-74.

Ijland MM, Pereira RR, Cornelissen EA (2008). Incidence of late vitamin K deficiency bleeding in newborns in the Netherlands in 2005: evaluation of the current guideline. European Journal of Pediatrics 167(2): 165-69.

Israels LG and Israels ED (1995). Observations on vitamin K deficiency in the fetus and newborn: has nature made a mistake? Seminars in Thrombosis and Hemostasis. 21(4): 357-63.

Israels LG, Israels ED and Saxena SP (1997). The riddle of vitamin K1 deficit in the newborn. Seminars in Perinatology. 21(1): 90-6.

Kay P (2000). The Vitamin K Controversy. Birth Gazette 16(2):19-21.

Khambalia AZ, Roberts CL, Bowen JR *et al* (2012). Maternal and infant characteristics by mode of vitamin K prophylaxis administration. Journal of Paediatrics and Child Health 48(8): 665-68.

Kojima T, Asoh M, Yamaqaki N *et al* (2004). Vitamin K concentrations in the maternal milk of Japanese women. Acta Paediatrica 93(4): 457-63.

Koklu E, Taskale T, Koklu S *et al*, (2014). Anaphylactic shock due to vitamin K in a newborn and review of literature. The Journal of Maternal-Fetal and Neonatal Medicine 27(11): 1180-81.

Laubscher B, Banziger O, Schubiger G *et al* (2013). Prevention of vitamin K deficiency bleeding with three oral mixed micellar phylloquinone doses: results of a 6-year (2005-2011) surveillance in Switzerland. European Journal of Pediatrics 172(3): 357-60

Lehmann, J (1944). Vitamin K as a prophylactic in 13,000 infants. Lancet. 243: 493–94

Lippi G and Franchini M (2011). Vitamin K in neonates: facts and myths. Blood Transfusion. 9(1): 4–9.

McKinney PA, Juszczak E, Findlay E *et al* (1998). Case-control study of childhood leukaemia and cancer in Scotland: findings for neonatal IM vitamin K. British Medical Journal 316: 173-77.

McNinch A, Busfield A, Tripp J (2007). Vitamin K deficiency bleeding in Great Britain and Ireland: British Paediatric Surveillance Unit Surveys, 1993 94 and 2001-02. Archives of Disease in Childhood 92(9): 759-66.

McNinch A (2010). Vitamin K deficiency bleeding: early history and recent trends in the United Kingdom. Early Human Development 86(1 suppl):63-65.

McNinch AW, Tripp JH (1991). Haemorrhagic disease of the newborn in the British Isles. British Medical Journal 303:1105-09

Neiger D (2004). Choices and changes Midwifery Matters 102:13-15.

Nishiguchi T, Saga K, Sumimoto K *et al*. (1996). Vitamin K prophylaxis to prevent neonatal vitamin K deficient intracranial haemorrhage in Shizuoka prefecture. British Journal of Obstetrics and Gynaecology 103(11): 1078-84.

Parker L, Cole M, Craft AW *et al* (1998), Neonatal vitamin K administration and childhood cancer in the north of England. British Medical Journal 316: 189-93.

Passmore SJ, Draper G, Brownbill P *et al* (1998). Ecological studies of relation between hospital policies on neonatal vitamin K administration and subsequent occurrence of childhood cancer British Medical Journal 316: 184-89.

Phillippi JC, Holley SL, Morad A *et al* (2016). Prevention of Vitamin K Deficiency Bleeding. Journal of Midwifery and Women's Health. 61(5): 632-636.

Pilcher E and Pilcher L (2008). The neonatal coagulation system and the vitamin K deficiency bleeding - a mini review. Wiener

Medizinische Wochenschrift 158: 385-95.

Politi MC, Jones KM and Philpott SE (2017). The Role of Patient Engagement in Addressing Parents' Perceptions About Immunizations. Journal of the American Medical Association. Published online June 22, 2017. doi:10.1001/jama.2017.7168

Puckett RM, Offringa M (2002). Prophylactic vitamin K for vitamin K deficiency bleeding in neonates (Cochrane Review). In: The Cochrane Library, Issue 4 2002. Oxford: Update Software.

Reed R and Johnson-Cash J (2016). The Human Microbiome: considerations for pregnancy, birth and early mothering. www.midwifethinking.com/2016/04/13/the-human-microbiome-considerations-for-pregnancy-birth-and-early-mothering/

Robertshawe B (2009). How did you prescribe vitamin K (phytomenadione) today? Midwifery News (New Zealand College of Midwives) 55:35.

Roche Pharmaceuticals (2015). Product Information: Konakion MM Paediatric 2 mg/0.2 ml.
www.medicines.org.uk/emc/medicine/1699

Roman E, Fear NT, Ansell P et al. (2002). Vitamin K and childhood cancer: analysis of individual patient data from six case-control studies. British Journal of Cancer 86(1): 63-69.

Sankar MJ, Chandrasekaran A, Kumar P et al (2016). Vitamin K prophylaxis for prevention of vitamin K deficiency bleeding: a systematic review. Journal of Perinatology 36 Suppl 1:S29-35.

Schulte R, Jordan LC, Morad A et al (2014). Rise in late onset VKDB in young infants because of omission or refusal of prophylaxis at birth. Pediatric Neurology. 50(6): 564-68.

Shearer MJ, Rahim S, Barkhan P et al (1982). Plasma vitamin K1 in mothers and their newborn babies. Lancet. 1982(2): 460–63.

Shearer MJ (2009). Vitamin K deficiency bleeding (VKDB) in early infancy. Blood Reviews 23(2): 49-59.

Slattery JM (1994). Why we need a clinical trial for vitamin K. British Medical Journal 308: 908-910.

Strehle EM, Howey C, Jones R (2010). Evaluation of the acceptability of a new oral vitamin K prophylaxis for breastfed infants. Acta Paediatrica 99(3): 379-83.

Sutherland JM, Glueck HI, Gleser G (1967). Hemorrhagic disease of the newborn. Breastfeeding as a necessary factor in the pathogenesis. American Journal of Disease in Childhood 113(5): 524–33.

Sutor AH (2003). New aspects of vitamin K prophylaxis. Seminars in Thrombosis and Hemostasis 29(4): 373-76.

Tandoi F, Mosca F, Agosti M (2005). Vitamin K prophylaxis: leaving the old route for the new one? Acta Paediatrica 94(suppl 449): 125-28.

Thomas MW, Gebara BM (2004). Difficulty breathing. Clinical Pediatrics. 43(5): 499-502.

Townsend CW (1894) The hemorrhagic disease of the newborn. Archives of Pediatrics 11: 559-65.

van Winckel M, De Bruyne R, Van de Velde S *et al* (2009). Vitamin K, an update for the paediatrician. European Journal of Pediatrics 168(2): 127-34.

Vietti TJ, Murphy TP, James JA *et al* (1960). Observations on the prophylactic use of vitamin K in the newborn infant. Journal of Pediatrics 56: 343–46.

von Kries R, Hanawa Y (1993). Neonatal vitamin K prophylaxis. Report of Scientific and Standardization Subcommittee on Perinatal Haemostasis. Thrombosis and Haemostasis 69: 293-95.

von Kries R (1998). Neonatal vitamin K prophylaxis; the Gordian knot still awaits untying. British Medical Journal 316: 161-62.

von Kries R (1999). Oral versus intramuscular phytomenadione: safety and efficacy compared. Drug Safety 21: 1-6.

Warren M, Miller A, Traylor J *et al* (2013). Late vitamin K deficiency bleeding in infants whose parents declined vitamin K prophylaxis—Tennessee, 2013. Morbidity and Mortality Weekly Report 62(45): 901.

Whitfield MF, Salfield SAW (1980). Accidental Administration of Syntometrine in Adult Dosage to the Newborn. Archives of Disease in Childhood 55, 68-70.

WHO. Guideline: Delayed umbilical cord clamping for improved maternal and infant health and nutrition outcomes. Geneva, World Health Organization; 2014. www.who.int/nutrition/publications/guidelines/cord_clamping/en/

Wickham S (2000). Vitamin K: a flaw in the blueprint? Midwifery Today (56): 39-41.

Wickham S (2003). Vitamin K and the newborn. AIMS: London.

Wickham S (2013). Revisiting vitamin K and the newborn: what have we learned in a decade? Essentially MIDIRS 4(7): 17-23.

Zipursky A (1996). Vitamin K at birth. British Medical Journal 313:179.

Printed in Poland
by Amazon Fulfillment
Poland Sp. z o.o., Wrocław